"Grounded in science and clinical expertise, this workbook offers paren[illegible] to support their LGBTQ+ child. The authors thoughtfully address pressing questions and common challenges in parenting LGBTQ+ youth with clarity and compassion. This workbook is an excellent companion for therapy, parent support groups, or independent use."

Em Matsuno, *PhD, Assistant Professor of Counselling Psychology at Arizona State University and creator of the Parent Support Program, an online program for parents and caregivers of trans and nonbinary youth*

"This workbook offers tools, supported by research, to help parents or guardians build stronger relationships and affirming families with their LGBTQ+ child or youth. Filled with structured activities that foster personal reflection and skill building. Of note, is its emphasis on acknowledging parents' personal values, belief systems, and emotional reactions."

Catherine Grus, *PhD, Chief Psychologist Officer, National Register of Health Service Psychologists, Washington DC*

"This workbook beautifully translates the best clinical knowledge into practical, heartfelt guidance for the people who matter most: parents. As a clinical psychologist, I know that this kind of affirming support is the foundation for a child's well-being. It is an essential tool for any family committed to raising a happy, healthy, and resilient LGBTQ+ child."

Nick Grant, *PhD, ABPP, Past President, GLMA: Health Professionals Advancing LGBTQ+ Equality*

PARENTING LGBTQ+ YOUTH

This compassionate guide helps parents examine and transform their approach to raising LGBTQ+ youth through thoughtful explorations of personal values, societal expectations, and the power of loving support.

Using the authors' LOVE framework (Looking at Our Values and Expectations), this engaging workbook helps parents understand their vital role in their LGBTQ+ child's identity development and well-being. Drawing on extensive clinical work, research, and personal experience, it offers insights and strategies to affirm and support parents as they navigate the challenges and joys of raising children to be their authentic selves. This book is divided into six modular chapters; each one explores an important theme, experience, and/or assumption with tools for readers navigating these critical stages in their parenting journey. Each activity is based on scientifically proven ways of boosting self-understanding, self-confidence, emotion regulation, and relationship quality. Chapters invite opportunities for learning and self-reflection and offer tools to promote healthy conversations and advocacy in various social contexts. At the end of this book, parents will have gained an invaluable set of tools for developing deeper insights and empathy for their LGBTQ+ child.

Parenting LGBTQ+ Youth is designed for readers in all stages of their parenting journey. It is an essential guide for parents, caregivers, and family members committed to active allyship and support of the LGBTQ+ youth in their lives.

Douglas Knutson (he/him), PhD, LHSP, ABPP, is Counseling Psychology Program Training Director and Associate Professor at Oklahoma State University, USA.

Kim Shenold (she/her), BA, is Transitional Living and Intervention Programs Coordinator at Payne County Youth Services, Inc., where she provides a wide range of outreach, education, and group services.

Janet Fultz (she/her), NCC, MS, LPC-S, is Executive Director of Payne County Youth Services, Inc., and has served the Payne County area via clinical services, administration, outreach, and grant writing for more than 25 years.

PARENTING LGBTQ+ YOUTH

A Workbook for Building Affirming Families

Douglas Knutson, Kim Shenold
and Janet Fultz

Routledge
Taylor & Francis Group
NEW YORK AND LONDON

Designed cover image: Getty Images

First published 2027
by Routledge
605 Third Avenue, New York, NY 10158

and by Routledge
4 Park Square, Milton Park, Abingdon, Oxon, OX14 4RN

Routledge is an imprint of the Taylor & Francis Group, an informa business

ISBN: 978-1-041-15182-1 (hbk)
ISBN: 978-1-041-14590-5 (pbk)
ISBN: 978-1-003-67820-5 (ebk)

DOI: 10.4324/9781003678205

Typeset in Stone Serif
by Apex CoVantage, LLC

DEDICATIONS

Joint Dedication

To the sort of love only a parent can give. When we began this work, this book was titled Parenting by LOVE (Looking at Our Values and Expectations). We were drawn to this title for two reasons: 1. It gave readers an idea of how we would approach the topic of parenting queer youths, and 2. It highlighted the inherent aspect of parental love that requires one to repeatedly take stock in the "how" of parenting. That is, as children grow and learn, the ways we parent them must be reevaluated and often adjusted to meet their new and ongoing needs, and to clear mental space from those needs that have been met. We also believe that, when we love another person, we must pull from the best version of ourselves, and we must open up space for the people we love to become the best versions of themselves. At its core, building an affirming family based on love is about finding yourself . . . and being found by others. It is a process of seeing and being seen; it is a journey that expands your values, heals your expectations, and embraces the messiness of life. This book is for the families who work hard to LOVE and the children who will be healed when their families define themselves, not by perfection, but by bravery. This book is for the often-unseen heroes who dare to parent by LOVE.

Douglas' Dedication

To Marsha P. Johnson, Allen Ginsberg, Harvey Fierstein, and all the queer heroes who dared to shine bright enough to light a path forward for generations of queer people, cast out of their families and communities. This book is an attempt to translate their brave calls for pride, authenticity, and radical self-acceptance into actionable steps for parents. It is written with the awareness that queer poetry can soothe an aching soul and instill hope in a lonely queer heart, but nothing can replace the hug of a proud parent. This book is a hug, a dream, and an invitation to keep the legacy of our queer ancestors alive.

Kim's Dedication

To my mother and her veiled love of whimsey; she nourished my creativity and independence, and she taught me to, unapologetically, be myself.

To my husband, without whom I would have no soft place to land when falling backward, as one does from time to time.

To my son, for being fierce in the face of adversity and more courageous than I ever expected. Still, he grounds me in childlike wonder and reminds me to bend, rather than break.

Janet's Dedication

It is my honor to dedicate this workbook to those whom we hope it will serve. It is further my honor to dedicate this work to those who helped me to understand the justice of this effort to support children and youth of the LGBTQ+ population. Much hope is found in my children, grandchildren, and LGBTQ+ family members, and the clients from whom I have learned so much. To my co-authors, you are the reason this work exists. I am grateful for you.

CONTENTS

PREFACE

It is my sincere pleasure, both personally and professionally, to have played a small part in the visioning and direction of this important resource for parents and guardians of LGBTQ+ children and youth. My co-authors and I bring our personal and professional perspective and expertise to this subject matter. We have all fought for, advocated for, provided services to, questioned the injustice for, and cried for someone in our professional or personal circles who has been harmed based solely on their exploration and understanding of who they each are regarding their sexual orientation and gender identity. We have each questioned the why's, turned to the research, and perhaps, most importantly, listened to the individual stories of our clients and family members as they each shared the joys and sorrows of their own lived experience as members of the LGBTQ+ population.

Across my 26-year counseling career, I have witnessed the ever-present pendulum swing in social, political, religious, and relational norms and their impact on individuals, families, and systems. As a licensed professional counselor and executive director of a non-profit, youth services agency in rural Oklahoma, I have been able to observe, design, and implement programs and interventions in emergency youth shelter systems, school-based and community-based mental health and substance abuse counseling, and through prevention, intervention, and advocacy programs. I have been able to work at state and local levels in education and advocacy.

I have found how very long it sometimes takes to move systems to even consider conversations, much less to act on strategies to enhance well-being for vulnerable children and youth. I have been ecstatic when successes and new interventions fall into place and when one can see the efforts creating real change and understanding. I have come to believe that most parents truly want the best for their child and that many of us need some additional tools to be the most effective we can be. I have sat with suicidal youth, with frightened parents, with abuse victims and trafficking survivors, and with children and youth who have lived safe lives with supportive parents and environments who still are in turmoil. I have witnessed healing, renewal, and joy among many.

Many years ago, I sat with parents (a cis, heterosexual man and woman), who pleaded with me to provide or refer them to conversion therapy. What struck me the most with that couple was their most sincere belief that providing their child with conversion therapy was the most loving and supportive thing they could do for their child. There was no judgment from them toward the child. Their pain was raw and palpable, their love for their child obvious, and their despair hung heavily in the room. As I tried to explain why that was not something I could or would do (how it was not ethical and what the science behind conversion therapy was), their hopelessness became almost unbearable. The lack of understanding of sexual orientation and gender identify development (and the potential power of the positive impact they could make) was profound and has been a professional experience that has moved me to continued advocacy for this population. Being blessed with family members who are members of the LGBTQ+ population both began and has continued my desire to include this important work as a part of my professional career.

While these struggles are not unique to the LGBTQ+ population, generational dysfunction, mental health and substance use, self-harm, educational and economic challenges, runaway behavior, death by suicide, abuse, bullying, isolation, depression, incidence of being a victim of violence, social issues, and the risk of victimization occur at higher rates for our LGBTQ+ members of society than for other populations, not because they are inherently more prone to these challenges, but because of how society and its members are ignorant to their needs or, worse, cause intentional harm. Current changes in law and practice that are quickly removing protections and services for LGBTQ+ persons are on the top of mind for our youth and their families, and their hopelessness and helplessness seem to escalate daily.

Working much of my career in the youth services field, I can attest to the many layers in our work as we strive to meet the needs of the individual. We must also consider their status if the client is a minor, the impact and resources of the family, the school, educational needs, spiritual needs, safety needs, all in the context of the normal developmental stages that children and youth experience.

Let's face it, a teenager can, sometimes, be a challenge to any family. Yet we know those challenges are partly due to the rapidly expanding brain and neural pathways, which may lead to critical growth that will occur during this period. Developing into adulthood is not for the faint of heart, nor is being the parent or guardian of someone in that stage of life. All youth develop their understanding of identity across many domains and are influenced by many norms. As the pendulum has swung in these areas to challenge the long-held norms of many in our society, it is my and my co-authors' belief that parents, mental health workers, educators, medical professionals, faith leaders, politicians, and more have a wonderful opportunity to help our children and youth have a "nova moment," exploding like a new star that suddenly becomes much brighter than it previously was, where it will shine for years. Think of it: Young people who are supported across their sexual orientation and gender identities to shine and share their light with their families and with the world; who are encouraged in their bravery, resilience, and compassion to be true to themselves, whatever that looks like, and to extend that privilege to those around them.

It is our hope that your use of this workbook (whether you are a parent or guardian, a family member, educator, or mental health provider, or through whatever dynamic you interact with LGBTQ+ young people) will assist you in developing a deeper understanding of your own perspective, allow you to challenge thoughts and ideas that might inhibit your support of the LGBTQ+ community, provide usable tools for effective and compassionate communication, and help that important task of children and youth developing into adulthood be more smooth and rewarding while creating space for a more positive, intentional relationship to flourish.

A word of clarification and caution: My co-authors and I do not presume to know, nor do we need to know, how you feel about the societal, religious, political, or other dynamics that surround this topic for you, your child, or your environment (however we welcome that sharing if you so desire). We come to this task with the desire to meet each of you where you are on your journey. We do not intend to judge actions, words, or beliefs. We do hope to share with you research-based concepts, models, activities, and actions you may wish to take to build your relationship with your child or youth, to help them be safe and to move into a future you and they will be a part of, with resiliency, joy, skills, and a belief in themself and in you.

As you move through this workbook, from Starting Out, to Looking Inward, to Coming Out and Advocacy, you will be given ideas and solid strategies based in scientific research that we firmly believe will help you in your parenting and relationship quest. The evolution of this workbook, growing from requests from parents in our communities for more skills in supporting their LGBTQ+ children, has included multiple rounds of focus groups and input from parents and guardians just like you. We look forward to your experience with this workbook. We wish for you insight and skills that enhance your parenting experience and for positive outcomes for you and your child. May you and your children find your way to the bright, nova-like light that shines when families are empowered to be who they are without judgment.

Janet Fultz, NCC, MS, LPC-S

ABOUT THE AUTHORS

Douglas Knutson (he/him), PhD, LHSP, ABPP, is Myron Ledbetter/Bob Lemon Counseling Psychology Diversity Associate Professor and Director of Training for the Counseling Psychology program in the School of Community Health Sciences, Counseling and Counseling Psychology at Oklahoma State University. He is the director of the Health, Education, and Rural Empowerment (HEaRE) Lab and recipient of the 2022 AMSA/GLMA LGBTQ Health Achievement Award. Douglas' recent book *Counseling in a Gender Expansive World: Resources to Support Therapeutic Practice* was the recipient of a 2023 American Psychological Association (APA) Division 44 Distinguished Book Award. He is the recipient of the 2023 APA Excellence in Rural Psychology Award and the 2023 Judy E. Hall Early Career Psychologist Award. Douglas is a member of the APA (Divisions 17, 35, and 44), associate editor for the *Journal of Rural Mental Health*, director of the APA Division 17 Communications and Technology Board, and Vice Chair of the APA Committee on Rural Health.

Kim Shenold (she/her), BA, is the Transitional Living and Intervention Programs Coordinator at Payne County Youth Services (PCYS), Inc., in Stillwater, Oklahoma. Kim facilitates a variety of programs at PCYS, including parenting groups, life skills groups, suicide prevention trainings, and staff trainings. Kim pulls from her experience as a parent educator, writer, ally to the LGBTQ+ community, and the parent of a gender-diverse teenager to bring education and awareness to parents and caregivers of LGBTQ+ youth throughout Payne County, Oklahoma, and beyond.

Janet Fultz (she/her), NCC, MS, LPC-S, is the Executive Director of Payne County Youth Services, Inc., and has provided supervision, clinical services, outreach, group facilitation, curriculum design, and grant writing expertise to the surrounding community for more than 25 years. Janet has devoted her career to supporting resilience and health in families, providing clinical training for counseling students at Oklahoma State University, and clinical supervision for those pursuing licensure. Janet has devoted significant time and provided critical assistance to non-profit excellence, systems design, advocacy, legislative impact, and community awareness and support to improve accessibility of services and positive outcomes for children, youth, and families facing emotional, behavioral, mental health, and substance use challenges. She has been intentional about creating space in her professional career and workplaces to address and advocate for the unique needs of the youth LGBTQ+ community. Her work is informed by current science, best practices, and an applied understanding of clinical excellence.

ACKNOWLEDGMENTS

The authors would like to thank Justin Shenold for creating all of the original artwork in this workbook. They are also grateful for the time and energy Nathan Armstrong put into reviewing and formatting the chapters. Last, but not least, they are deeply thankful for the parents, Oklahoma State University Counseling Psychology doctoral students, and queer community members who made this workbook possible.

Development of this workbook was financially supported by the National Register of Health Service Psychologists through the Judy E. Hall Early Career Psychologist Award presented to Dr. Douglas Knutson in 2023. This work was also supported by Douglas Knutson's Myron Ledbetter/Bob Lemon Counseling Psychology Diversity Professorship. Payne County Youth Services staff were key partners in the development of the materials presented in this text.

INTRODUCTION

Welcome to the Parenting LGBTQ+ Youth workbook. We are excited that you decided to give this book a try. We hope you find this workbook a welcome tool for you as you explore your important role in the life of an LGBTQ+ young person. Whether you are the biological parent, foster parent, guardian, or simply the primary caregiver to a child or teen who identifies as LGBTQ+, you are in the right place.

Origins of the Workbook

This workbook grew out of a rural health initiative between a large state university and a rural-facing clinic in the heartland of the United States. It was developed in the period after the death of Nex Benedict and at a time when parents were experiencing increasing backlash for supporting their trans and nonbinary children. At the time this book was published, legal and social pressures were continuing to increase on parents, but especially caregivers for rural LGBTQ+ youth. In many ways, this book is our contribution to the fight to support, empower, and stand with families who are determined to show up for LGBTQ+ youth despite the legal and social risks involved in doing so.

We share this context because the first iteration of this workbook was titled "Parenting by LOVE," and LOVE stood for "Looking at our Values and Expectations." The title had a deep meaning for us because it acknowledged that this project was a labor of love and it pointed to the core assumptions of this project. Based on years of research, practice, and community-engaged work, we know that many of the limitations faced by LGBTQ+ youth stem from misunderstandings, limited expectations, and a lack of experience. When parents and guardians examine their expectations and values, they often find that supporting their LGBTQ+ child is not at odds with their worldview. On the contrary, affirming their child is consistent with their identity and goals as a parent.

After we developed this workbook, we shared it with community partners and gathered feedback about ways to make it better and more closely aligned with the needs of rural communities. Then we invited groups of parents to engage with the workbook in educational settings. We discovered that the workbook offered encouragement, guidance, and insights to parents that were reassuring and healing. They discovered a community of parents who were experiencing many of the same challenges, breakthroughs, and heartwarming moments with their own LGBTQ+ youth. Those groups, and the families who were brave enough to attend them, inspired us to make this work more broadly available.

As you start this journey toward parenting by LOVE, we want you to know that you are not alone. A growing number of teens across the United States are coming out to their parents/caregivers as lesbian, gay, bisexual, transgender, and so on (LGBTQ+). In 2020, about 9.5% of the U.S. population between ages 13–17 identified as LGBTQ+, and nearly 1 in 4 high schoolers (in grades 9–12) identified with a category other than heterosexual (Centers for Disease Control and Prevention, 2024; Williams Institute, 2020). You may feel isolated or unique in the current sociopolitical and legal climate, but nothing could be further from the truth. You are part of a large and growing segment of society, you are one of many grounded, productive, caring people, determined to love an LGBTQ+ child. You are in good company.

Of course, we can tell you until we are blue in the face that you are part of a large community, but that is easier to think about than to feel. In reality, parenting an LGBTQ+ child can feel scary and isolating, especially if you do not know other LGBTQ+ people or families in your community. Soon after your child comes out, your head may fill up with questions like, "What will my parents think if they find out?", "How will people at church react?" or "Is this all my fault?". Lots of parents think these thoughts (Birnkrant & Przeworski, 2017; Bull & D'Arrigo-Patrick, 2018) and that is another reason we created this workbook.

The Importance of Families

It is true that this book was a labor of love that grew out of tragedy and a desire to support parents, but it also grew out of an awareness of the central and crucial role that families play in the lives of LGBTQ+ youth and adults. The simple fact is that there is no replacement for support from our families of origin. You may be aware that many LGBTQ+ people create "chosen families" and find other creative sources of support, but researchers suggest that chosen families simply are not replacements for parental support (Milton & Knutson, 2023).

You are an essential part of your child's success in this world. Your involvement in your child's life does not make them LGBTQ+, but it can help to reduce risk factors, increase or maintain safety, and help your child succeed in life as a healthy, whole, and fulfilled human being (Tate & Patterson, 2019). That is a liberating reality. You did not break your child, but you can help them thrive. This workbook is designed, in part, to help parents shift from a mindset that asks "How can I fix my LGBTQ+ child?" to a mindset that poses the question, "How can I help my LGBTQ+ child thrive?"

The Journey Ahead

You may be opening this workbook for the first time because your child just came out to you as LGBTQ+ and you don't know what to do. Or maybe your child told you they were LGBTQ+ years ago, and you are now able to engage with their unique identity. One thing is for sure, the way you relate to your child will change over time (Abreu et al., 2020). That means that this workbook will have a different meaning and a different impact each time you open it. We encourage you to view it as a resource or a journey that you can return to, update, and reflect on now and in the future.

When you were a child, you might have had a baby book (or "growing up book") in which your parent could keep a record of your first word, first steps, and so on. You might view this workbook as a way to document your own growth with your child or as a "growing up book" of sorts in which you can record, revisit, revise, and add to your memories, musings, and breakthroughs on your journey toward LOVE. Regardless of where you are on your journey toward accepting and affirming your LGBTQ+ child, we hope this workbook will help.

This workbook uses a trauma-informed, self-exploratory approach to strengthening the connections and relationships in your family. We mentioned that early drafts of this workbook were used in a group setting, and it can be a very useful tool for PFLAG meetings, clinicians, and community centers. Those groups helped us refine, focus, and hone the materials, but this workbook was always meant for rural and remote families who might not have the option to access group therapy. You will notice ways the materials can be adapted for use with groups, but if you are working through this material at home or on your own, you can rest assured, this book is for you.

Next Steps

Thank you for picking up this book and committing to the difficult and rewarding journey ahead. On the pages that follow, you will find a series of worksheets designed to help you process through and examine your identity and your future as the parent of an LGBTQ+ child.

We recommend starting at the beginning of this book and completing each chapter in order. It is possible to use the workbook as a source of worksheets and activities in a clinical setting, but each chapter is designed to build on the insights gained from the chapter before it. Extracting individual chapters may interrupt the intended learning process, and clinicians who use the content out of sequence should be prepared to fill in learning gaps and ensure participants are prepared for the activities they are asked to complete.

The workbook is also designed to be completed in six weeks, either in a group format or as a tool for self-study. Engaging with the workbook in this limited time span helps readers stay on track and can further ensure that the content and progress readers make stays fresh in their minds. In group settings, we generally recommend keeping class sizes to 5–10 parents and running groups from 1.5–2 hours. For self-study, we suggest working through a chapter a week and one subsection each day. Instead of playing on your phone or watching TV in bed before you go to sleep, try working through a subsection or worksheet before dozing off to sleep.

Of course, there is no right way to complete the workbook, and it is best not to let the perfect be the enemy of the good. In other words, if you complete it all in one day or take a year to get through the chapters, the most important thing is for you to learn, grow, and gain confidence. To facilitate that growth, each chapter includes a review of key research, engaging activities, case examples, and opportunities to reflect.

- Chapter 1 offers the opportunity to explore your boundaries, needs, and rights as a participant in this workshop.
- In Chapter 2, you will learn current terminology, concepts, and facts surrounding the identities and development of LGBTQ+ kids.
- Chapter 3 provides worksheets to help you explore your own gender and affectional journey as a way to better understand your child's experiences and needs.
- In Chapter 4, you will reflect on your child's unique development and growth from birth to present.
- Chapter 5 provides space to explore social, medical, and other coming out processes that your child may go through as they grow toward adulthood.
- In Chapter 6, you will identify ways to advocate for your child and other LGBTQ+ youth.

Preparing for Success

This learning process may be hard, frustrating, or even unpleasant at times, but the journey is worth it. As you work through this workbook, we encourage you to use self-compassion, a technique proven to help reduce self-judgment and distress (Neff, 2011). For example, imagine how you might respond to a close friend who is in a similar situation. Chances are you would support your friend, try to understand their struggles, and encourage them to stay strong. We invite you to extend that same compassion to yourself.

There are a lot of outside pressures on parents that came up in our early work on this book. For example:

- There are people who judge parents for not rejecting or trying to fix their LGBTQ+ children.
- There are people who judge parents for not immediately understanding and unreservedly supporting their LGBTQ+ children.
- There are children who express frustration toward their parents for not "getting it."

As you engage with this workbook, we hope you will do your best to set those voices and outside judgments aside. When you read these pages and engage with these activities, you have permission to be you. You can write your thoughts, acknowledge your feelings, and celebrate your bravery. In other words, there is no right way to complete this workbook. This is your space and your journey.

The fact that you are engaging with this workshop is evidence that you are brave and determined and that you deeply love your child. We hope you will keep that love in mind as you progress through these pages. This workbook is based on the most recent research and scholarship available. If you are interested in a list of resources, please see the bibliography at the end of the workbook. Now let's get started on this journey of LOVE.

References

Abreu, R. L., Gonzalez, K. A., Rosario, C. C., Pulice-Farrow, L., & Rodríguez, M. M. D. (2020). "Latinos have a stronger attachment to the family": Latinx fathers' acceptance of their sexual minority children. *Journal of GLBT Family Studies, 16*(2), 192–210. https://doi.org/10.1080/1550428X.2019.1672232

Birnkrant, J. M., & Przeworski, A. (2017). Communication, advocacy, and acceptance among support-seeking parents of transgender youth. *Journal of Gay & Lesbian Mental Health, 21*(2), 132–153. https://doi.org/10.1080/19359705.2016.1277173

Bull, B., & D'Arrigo-Patrick, J. (2018). Parent experiences of a child's social transition: Moving beyond the loss narrative. *Journal of Feminist Family Therapy, 30*(3), 170–190. https://doi.org/10.1080/08952833.2018.1448965

Centers for Disease Control and Prevention. (2024). *Youth Risk Behavior Survey data summary & trends report: 2013–2023*. U.S. Department of Health and Human Services. https://www.cdc.gov/yrbs/dstr/index.html

Conron, J. K. (2020, September). *LGBT youth population in the United States*. Williams Institute. https://williamsinstitute.law.ucla.edu/publications/lgbt-youth-pop-us/

Milton, C., & Knútson, D. (2021). Family of origin, not chosen family, predicts psychological health in a LGBTQ+ sample. *Psychology of Sexual Orientation and Gender Diversity*. https://doi.org/10.1037/sgd0000531

Neff, K. (2011). *Self-compassion: The proven power of being kind to yourself*. William Morrow.

Tate, D. P., & Patterson, C. J. (2019). Sexual orientation, relationships with parents, stress, and depressive symptoms among adults. *Journal of GLBT Family Studies, 15*(3), 256–271. https://doi.org/10.1080/1550428X.2018.1486263

CHAPTER 1

BEGINNING YOUR JOURNEY TOWARD BUILDING AN AFFIRMING FAMILY

Starting Out

Before starting any big journey that involves the potential for changes to your thoughts, feelings, and behaviors, it is important to set a plan and clarify your goals (Epton et al., 2017). You may have experienced going on a poorly planned hike at some point in your life. If not, you can at least imagine starting up a mountain feeling hydrated and optimistic at the beginning of a beautiful day, but after hours of climbing, the newness wears off. Your single bottle of water runs dry, and your stomach starts to rumble. You turn back early out of fear that you will go too far without the food and water needed to make it back to the trailhead safely.

Similarly, goals can be most effective when they are challenging and are shared with others (Epton et al., 2017). We want you to be able to complete the journey through this workbook safely, so we will start out by making sure you have the tools and resources necessary to keep going when the going gets tough. We also feel it's important to be able to look back and see how far you've come (Hawkins et al., 2004), so our first activity is designed to help us benchmark our starting point.

The next step is to complete a therapeutic contract or a learning contract that will help set you up for success (e.g., Wilson & Murrell, 2011). Learning contracts, similar to a trail map, clearly spell out the commitments, responsibilities, and needs you bring with you as you start an educational journey. You need to commit to the hike before you start it (Urmanche et al., 2019).

After completing your learning contract, you will declare your rights and freedoms as a parent. It can be empowering and energizing to know you are equal to the task ahead and properly prepared for the trek. Establishing your list of rights reminds you that you have the strength, capacity, and resources to see this through (Lannin et al., 2019).

Last of all, you will set a plan for what to do when the journey gets too hard. When the incline is steep or you fall and skin your knee, it can be easy to regret the trip entirely and want to turn back. Time spent in an unfamiliar wilderness or walking uncharted territory can be downright terrifying. It may be comforting to know you have a safety plan, that you have a satellite phone, so to speak, that you can pull out of your bag and call a friend for help when you become most afraid or feel you are alone (see Rogers et al., 2022).

Before we begin the first activity, we want to acknowledge it can be challenging to identify and explore thoughts and ideas that may challenge our current way of thinking or that ask us to acknowledge biases we may hold that create conflict with people we love. At any time during your journey through this workbook, you are encouraged to take a break, reach out to a trusted friend or family member, or seek professional help and support when working with thoughts or ideas that cause you distress or discomfort. Remember, people have more success reaching important goals when they connect with others (Epton et al., 2017).

DOI: 10.4324/9781003678205-1

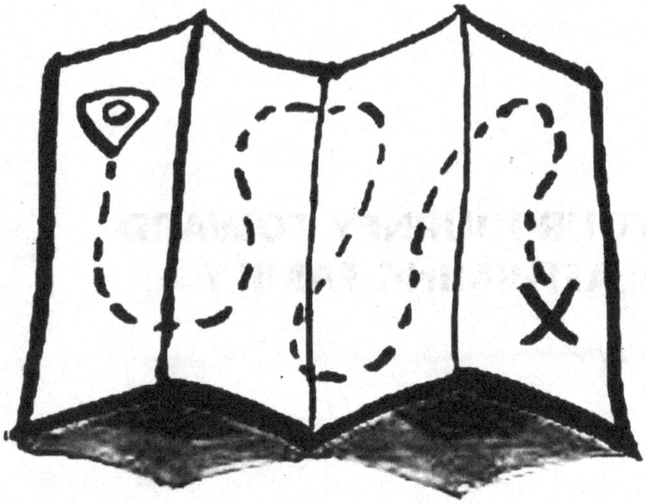

Image 1.1 The journey ahead.

We also want to reassure you that whatever you are feeling about this journey is valid and likely to change over time (Abreu et al., 2020). Some people will come to this work with a sense of optimism; they're experienced hikers and come ready or even excited for a new challenge! Some people will come to this work with a sense of anxiety or fear; they've never hiked before and are unsure what to pack or if their boots will hold up to the terrain; maybe they don't know how to decipher the trail map or where to even begin. Our goal is for experienced hikers and novices alike to reach the end of this journey safely and to find there that it was well worth the effort.

The journey ahead may appear challenging, and research demonstrates that engaging in interventions for caregivers of LGBTQ+ youth can also be rewarding (Austin et al., 2021). Reaching the top of the mountain gives you views, memories, and feelings of fulfillment you might never have experienced if not for the trek up. Having an LGBTQ+ child presents unique challenges, and it can also be rewarding and filled with joy and unique victories (Abreu et al., 2023). It can be tough to rethink values, explore different realities, and try out new ways of thinking. This chapter is designed to help you feel as safe and empowered as possible as you journey toward the powerful gift you receive when you love and affirm your LGBTQ+ child for who they are as a unique individual.

Step 1: Identifying Your Dreams

For this first activity, we ask that you take a moment to reflect on your early experiences as a parent. Close your eyes, if you like, and think back to your first visions about who your child might be as an adult when you first found out that you would be a parent or guardian. Feel free to jot down some preliminary thoughts that you will be able to further develop in the upcoming activity.

> Want to learn more about imaginary exercises as a therapeutic tool? Check out Appendix B: Activity 1 Scientific Basis for more on this topic.

Now think about the sorts of "plans" or expectations that popped into your mind. What is the common theme between the various hopes and dreams you have for your child? For example, did your thoughts center around:

- What will their future career be?
- Who will they marry?
- Where will they live?
- What level of education will they obtain and in what field?

For now, don't worry too much about how your teen would react to these "plans." There is no judgment here. Your dreams are valid, and they often drive your expectations for the future. For now, we just want you to explore what you thought life for your child would look like, especially as it relates to their relationships and life achievements. For example, when the doctor told you the sex of your unborn child, did you start planning future shopping trips with your daughter-in-law, or start exploring ways to get your child into law school?

When you are ready, transfer the ideas you jotted down (or saved in your brain) to Activity 1. You might have a lot to write down, but try sticking to the four strongest hopes, aspirations, or desires you had for your child. You may write down your thoughts or draw images that represent the dreams you have or had for your child before you learned of their LGBTQ+ identity.

As you work through this activity, remind yourself the following:

- My hopes and dreams for my child are born of love and caring. It is okay to grieve aspirations that may never be met.
- It is okay for my hopes and dreams for my child to change over time.
- It is okay if my hopes and dreams for my child are different from their hopes and dreams for themself.

If you need to in the future, feel free to come back to these statements. They can serve as an important reminder that growing and changing are integral parts of parenting, and that, if you find you've taken a misstep, it is okay to reevaluate your footing and try again. Change is part of life, and certainly part of relationships.

Activity 1 My Identity Dream for My LGBTQ+ Child

Please record the dream(s) you had for your LGBTQ+ teen, especially as they relate to relationships and life achievements.

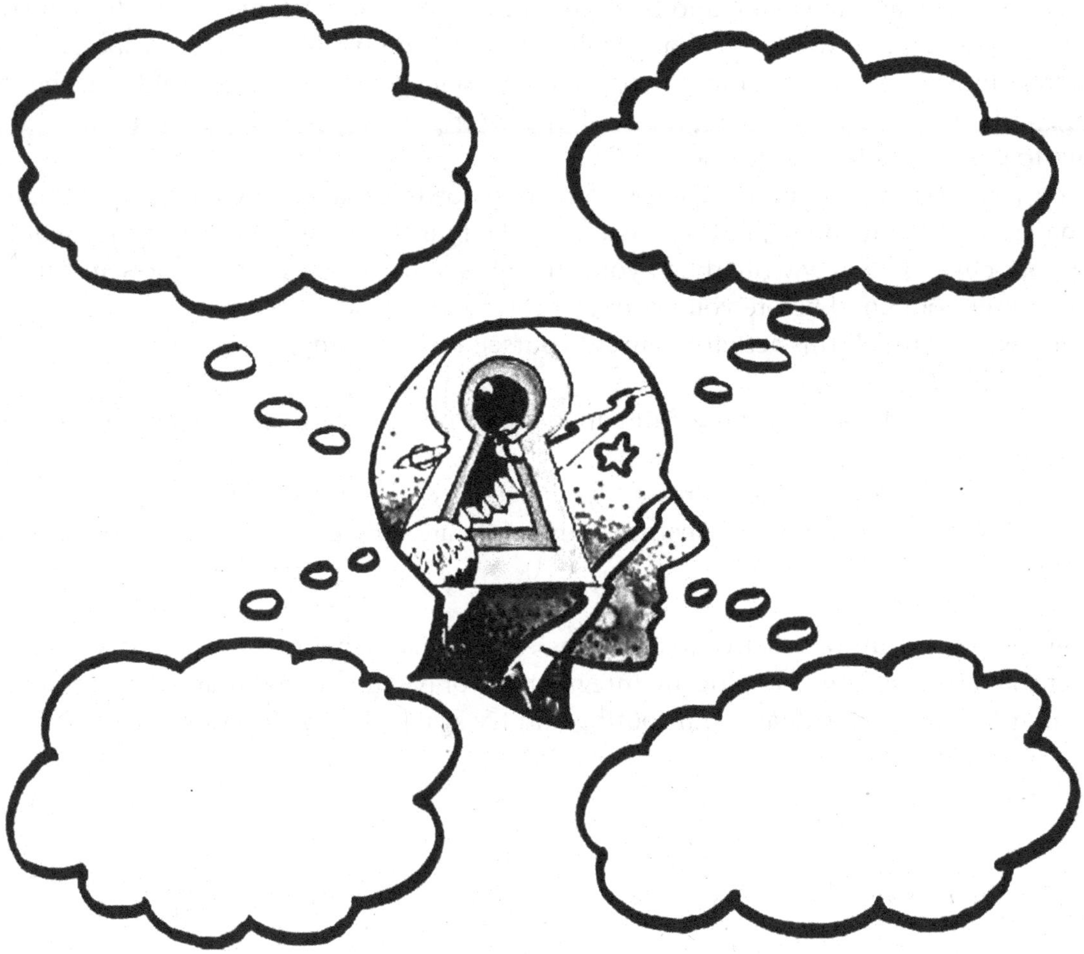

Image 1.2 Exploring your parenting dreams.

Step 2: Committing to Learn

Learning (like hiking) takes commitment. As experienced educators, we have seen the benefits of mentorship and teaching. We have watched students and parents make major breakthroughs and acquire skills that help them get to the next level of their careers, expand their futures, and open up new opportunities. At the same time, we have seen how challenging the learning process itself can be. Pushing your mind to develop new connections and branch new neurons is, quite frankly, hard work, and hard work is rarely pleasant.

As we stated earlier, you will be more likely to succeed if you set a plan and make a commitment (Wilson & Murrell, 2011).

> If you want to know more about goal setting, take a look at Appendix B: Activity 2 Scientific Basis.

Making a commitment, though, is only half of the story. You have probably agreed to a million little things throughout life, at least passively. When you are faced with adhering to social norms or being expected to "toe the line," it is sometimes easier to nod your head and go with the flow. You may feel you have to or fear potential outcomes of noncompliance.

This is not that kind of workbook. In fact, your work to affirm your LGBTQ+ child is revolutionary, voluntary, and intentional; we hope you feel empowered each time you return to these pages. The relationship between each LGBTQ+ teen and their parent or guardian is unique in many ways; therefore, we ask that you name *your* cause – the reason *you* are engaging with this workbook – so that when the terrain gets rocky, you can realign with your purpose and remember the commitment you made to yourself and to your LGBTQ+ teen. As you complete the activity for this section, please think deeply about what you are committing to do, acknowledge the intention it takes to engage in this process, and assert your cause.

There are two types of learning contracts in this workbook. If you are using this workbook for self-study, you can complete Activity 2.1. Because the workbook can be used to lead parenting groups and workshops, we included a learning contract that works better in group settings. If you are completing this in a group, you can skip to Activity 2.2. Regardless of how you complete the workbook, we designed the materials in this book so that you can return to them in years to come. In fact, when we piloted early versions of this workbook in parenting groups, we found that people responded to the materials differently, depending on where they were in their process of developing an affirming relationship with their child.

If you want, you can complete the workbook on your own now and then return to it in a few years and establish new goals. Likewise, if you are participating in this group a second time, feel free to use the blank learning contract to establish new goals. This is a tool for you that, like a baby book, keeps a record of one of the most important relationships in your life. We want this journey to be memorable and treasured for years to come.

Activity 2.1 Learning Contract for Self-Guided Study

I choose to engage in this work because ____

____

Through my experiences here, I hope to ____

____

I commit to approach this workbook with humility and openness.

I recognize that change is often uncomfortable and that it is an inevitable part of life and relationships.

I commit to treating myself with kindness and respect.

I commit to completing this work in a safe, affirming environment where I may engage with the material fully.

I agree to try to be forgiving of myself and others; mistakes are part of learning something new.

(Please use the space below for personal statements you may wish to add.)

____

____

____

I will work hard to remember why I choose to engage with this workbook, to prioritize this journey as an opportunity to grow and learn, and to reach out for help if I find myself overwhelmed or in distress.

______________________________ ______________

Signature Date

Activity 2.2 Learning Contract for Group Workshop

I choose to attend this workshop because ____

____

Through my experiences here, I hope to ____

____

I commit to approach this workshop with humility and openness.

I recognize that change is often uncomfortable and that it is an inevitable part of life and relationships.

As part of an open, community support group, I commit to treating fellow group members and leaders with kindness and respect.

I understand the importance of confidentiality and will not share information about others (including names and places of work or residence) who may attend this group with anyone outside of group. I understand that to break confidentiality may be a safety issue for group members.

I can expect group leaders to respect the confidentiality of all group members.

I can expect group leaders to maintain a safe, affirming environment where all group members may participate safely.

I agree to try to be forgiving of myself and others; mistakes are part of learning something new.

(Please use the space below for personal statements you may wish to add.)

____

____

____

I will work hard to remember why I choose to be here, to prioritize this journey as an opportunity to grow and learn, and to reach out for help if I find myself overwhelmed or in distress.

______________________________ ______________

Signature Date

Step 3: Embracing Your Rights

As you look at the road ahead, it can be helpful to claim your rights as a parent. These rights may include boundaries that you hold or permissions that you give yourself (Lannin et al., 2019). For example, you may wish to claim the right to "love my child deeply, even if I do not fully understand them," or to "advocate for my child, even if close family or friends don't agree." Maybe you want to claim the right to feel discomfort or confusion.

As you might have noticed, the rights you claim may run counter to messages you have heard in the past or core beliefs you hold about the quality of your parenting. For example, you may catch yourself believing, "I have to fully understand or 'get' my child in order to love them." Maybe your teen even said to you once, "You just don't get me!" as if that meant you had failed. This list of rights is yours, and you can use it to push back on some of the inaccurate messages you have picked up about your parenting.

Keep in mind that the rights you claim should not infringe on the rights of others (Saenz, 2015). For example, it would not be appropriate (or even possible) for you to claim that you have the right to "make others respect my child's pronouns," but it would be appropriate (and achievable) to say that you have the right to "ask/encourage others to respect my child's pronouns" or even to "discontinue contact with individuals who choose not to respect my child's pronouns."

There are two things to consider here. The first is that your rights statements may grow out of your goals. If your goals are measurable and achievable, they may help you draft concrete rights as well. The second consideration is safety. Your list of rights and goals may be aspirational, but they also need to be safety-informed and contextual. For example, correcting someone's pronoun use at a truck stop may be less safe than doing so at a family gathering. We encourage you to consider any safety issues that might be present for your child, yourself, or your family.

You may also want to consider your rights as an individual who is also a parent. What we mean here is, you have the right to feel the way you feel, even if it's not how you think a parent "should" feel (Jefferson et al., 2020). Again, outside messages and expectations can play into this process. For example, you may want to claim the right to "feel sad that my child doesn't want to have children of their own" or to "grieve the loss of the mother-daughter relationship I expected with my child" or even to "celebrate the new adventure of parenting a gender diverse person."

For more on grief and self-acceptance, check out Appendix B: Activity 3 Scientific Basis.

As you consider your rights as an individual, remember that feeling a certain way is always valid, and that sharing those feelings is a separate action (Egolf & Gold, 2023). In other words, while you have the right to feel sad or to grieve something you experience as a loss, it may not be helpful and could potentially be harmful to share all those feelings with your teen (D'amico et al., 2015; van Bergen et al., 2021). Before sharing potentially hurtful feelings with your teen, ask yourself if doing so is necessary and beneficial to both you and your relationship.

If you find that you would feel better to share feelings that your teen may find hurtful, we strongly encourage you to find someone else with whom you can share – a close friend or family member who will respect your confidentiality or a counselor or therapist may be able to help you process those feelings without hurting your child and the relationship you're working to improve (Ryan & Chen-Hayes, 2013).

Lastly, rest assured that your parenting list of rights is a living document – this means that you can change it at any time to better reflect current realities for yourself, your child, and your family. The rights you might have claimed as the parent of a toddler are likely quite different from the rights you feel should be claimed as the parent of a teenager. As your relationship with your LGBTQ+ teen evolves and develops, and as you grow and change as an individual, so may your parenting list of rights.

Activity 3 My Rights as a Parent

Please use the space below to record the parenting rights that are important for you.

I have the right to . . .

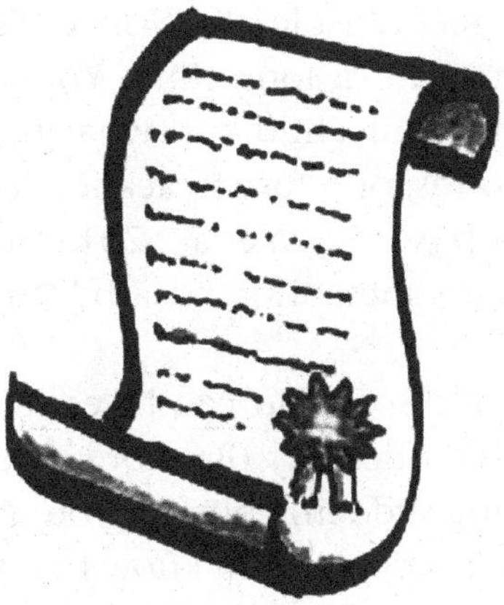

Image 1.3 Bill of rights.

- ____
- ____
- ____
- ____
- ____
- ____
- ____
- ____
- ____
- ____
- ____
- ____
- ____
- ____

Step 4: Planning for Hard Times

As we mentioned in the previous section, you may start to experience complex emotions that may include regret or pain as you progress through this workshop, deepen your bond with your child, and consider your values (Morgan et al., 2023). You may wish you could revisit ways you have acted in the past or feel remorse about the ways you yourself were treated when you were growing up. You may even hold the people closest to you (e.g., a parent, sibling, or partner) responsible for the ways they have shaped or restricted your beliefs and perspectives. These feelings can be hard to carry alone.

What's more, you might not feel terrible all at once. Feelings of remorse and sadness can build slowly and even escape your notice for a long time. Your experience may not be very unlike your child's in this regard. Think about your child and what it must be like for people to call them the wrong name, use the wrong pronouns, or refuse to acknowledge their identity over and over and over. Those individual hurts can build up (see Testa et al., 2015). Consider the phrase "death by a thousand papercuts" or to stick with our hiking metaphor, "death by a thousand bee stings" as a way to describe this dynamic.

Because individual moments of discomfort can be easier to ignore or minimize, it can be hard to identify when you are struggling emotionally (Balmores-Paulino, 2020). You may feel like your concerns are not valid or like something suddenly pushed you over the edge for no reason. As you embark on this journey, please take yourself seriously and know that your feelings are valid. It is okay to notice, validate, and process each "sting" along the way. They are all valid and, if they go unaddressed, they can fester.

As a parent, it is important to validate your feelings (Jefferson et al., 2020). Sometimes parents may not feel like they have permission to struggle. You may think that you must always be strong for your family. Or you may feel like you have to explain yourself to your child and share all your worries and concerns. Activity 4 is designed to help you identify when you might be distressed so that you can find ways to self-soothe or find the support you need.

> If at any time you find yourself in immediate need of care, you can call 988, the national suicide prevention and mental health crisis hotline, 911, or proceed to the nearest emergency room.

Noticing small, compounding stressors is a skill that does not come automatically for many people. You may need to monitor your emotions, identify ways your body responds to distress, and plan to check in with yourself at regular intervals. This section will walk you through some techniques you can use to identify and respond to distress by constructing a safety plan.

> For more information about safety plans, check out Appendix B: Activity 4 Scientific Basis.

First, think about experiences, conversations, or topics that are likely to cause you pain or discomfort – they may be papercuts that add up or major topics that you usually avoid.

Then, think about warning signs that you are getting upset. What usually happens when life gets to be too much (Rogers et al., 2022)? For example, your thoughts might get foggy, or your heart rate might speed up. On the next page, please record three warning signs. Next, think about activities you can do to calm yourself. What relaxes you the most? Please see the Calming Skills section at the back of the book for examples. Please record at least three self-soothing activities.

Sometimes, self-soothing is not enough, and you need to check in with someone (Rogers et al., 2022). Talking to someone else can help you identify warning signs that you may not see for yourself and calm you down when your regular self-soothing activities are not working. Think of an adult you trust that you could call in when you need support as a parent of an LGBTQ+ teen. You will be asked to write down your thoughts in Activity 4. You can refer to your plan at any time. It helps to commit to using your safety plan when you find yourself in distress (Kayman et al., 2015).

Activity 4 What to Do When It Gets Hard

What experiences, conversations, or topics are likely to cause you pain or discomfort – they may be papercuts that add up or major topics that you usually avoid?

- ____
- ____
- ____

What are some warning signs that you are getting upset?

- ____
- ____
- ____

What can you do to calm yourself? What relaxes you the most?

- ____
- ____
- ____

Who do you trust to support you when you get distressed? Please write down at least one contact person's name and phone number (not your child or your partner).

____

You may even find it helpful to take a picture of your Safety Plan to store on your phone for convenient access. Please read the commitment statement at the bottom of the page and sign and date your safety plan.

"I promise to pay attention to my needs and emotions while participating in this workshop. I will use the resources listed on this page to take care of myself and I will reach out for help if I need it."

____________________ ____________

Signature Date

Bringing It All Together

Congratulations on completing the first chapter of the workbook! If you have ever gone to therapy, you know the intake session is always the hardest part, and it often feels the least rewarding. Clients usually show up to therapy ready to work and then they find out they have to answer a bunch of questions as their therapist completes a very long intake form. If you picked up this book ready to get to work, we have good news for you: This book only gets better from here.

Still, just like any healing process, the first steps are some of the most important and we encourage you to acknowledge your accomplishment. Please refer to this chapter anytime you need support or to be reminded of your rights, responsibilities, and resources. As you reflect on your progress so far, take a moment to read over the following vignettes.

Each chapter includes an example of what engagement with the chapter might look like in real life. They are designed to supplement self-study for readers who are not completing this workbook in a group or with a clinician. The vignettes are made up and any resemblance to real people are coincidental. As you read each vignette in this book, you might reflect on how your experience has been similar and/or different and why that is the case.

Vignette 1: Mark

Mark is a 35-year-old father of two children (one 13-year-old daughter and one 15-year-old son) who lives in rural North Dakota. About a year ago, his 15-year-old son, Devin, came out to him as gay. At first, Mark did not know what to do. He believed that gay people "ended up that way" because they failed to bond with their fathers and over-identified with their mothers. Hoping that he could fix his son by "loving him more," Mark told Devin, "I completely support you and I am here for you. If you really believe this, you're going to have to tell your mom and grandparents." Mark never thought Devin would tell anybody else, but a week later, Devin told his mom, Sharon.

Sharon called Mark immediately after her conversation with Devin, sobbing so intensely that she could barely talk. She said she was afraid that Devin had AIDS, was on drugs, and was going to hell. Mark did his best to console his wife, but he found himself sharing her fears. For the next few months, Mark, Sharon, and Devin went through rupture and repair cycles marked by periods of silence, distancing, reconnection, yelling, and so on. Desperate for resources and a way forward, Mark found this workbook and asked Sharon to read it with him.

The first exercise was hard for Mark and Sharon. It caused them to relive their dreams for Devin. Sharon talked about how badly she wanted grandchildren and a daughter-in-law that she could do "girl stuff" with. Mark talked about feeling like he lost his only son. As they worked through the chapter, though, they were able to identify some of the feelings that were coming up and some of the signs they were in distress (Mark's heartrate kept spiking and Sharon kept getting tearful). They decided to embrace their reactions, and they decided they had the right to be unhappy, while also deeply loving their son. They also agreed to keep an eye on the "signs" that they were struggling, and they identified ways they could support each other.

Working with the workbook was hard for Mark in particular. He had been raised in an evangelical home and worked as a volunteer youth pastor at a local church. He knew the workbook was not aligned with his church's views, but he decided to commit to the materials and give the book a try. He particularly liked the way the workbook encouraged him to connect with his values, and he figured finding ways to love his son could look unique to him. If that was one of his core values, it would not hurt to explore it.

Vignette 2: Kerrie

Kerrie is a 38-year-old single mother who has always lived in the Southern Midwest. Kerrie considers herself open-minded and accepting of other people, especially given her socio-political surroundings. Kerrie had one child, Danice, from a marriage that didn't outlast the child's toddler years. Dani, the name he started using exclusively last year, told Kerrie a few months ago that he's not actually non-binary, he's trans. Kerrie remembers responding to this news favorably at first – she nodded in agreement and told Dani that she will always love him no matter what; she thinks she told him she would do her best to embrace his gender identity and may have said it would be difficult. . . . To be honest, it was kind of a whirlwind and the only thing she knows for sure is that she *wanted* to say the right things; she *wanted* Dani to feel safe with her no matter what.

Over the next few days, Kerrie began to realize she was terrified of how people might treat Dani, that she was scared of ongoing anti-trans legislation, and she was trying to figure out if their state had enacted punishments for affirming parents yet. Kerrie's mind was going in what felt like a million different directions, splintered into thoughts of protection, thoughts of "how to," and thoughts of "what if," just to name a few. Although she wouldn't admit it, Kerrie also wondered if Dani was just experiencing a phase, just trying on a new identity, and maybe this would all blow over before too long. One thing Kerrie knew, was that she felt lost; she wasn't sure who she could talk to, and she needed support.

When Kerrie signed up to take a free workshop for parents of LGBTQ+ teens in her community, she was nervous. Kerrie knew kids in her community felt safer now than they did when she was young because she's seen them wearing rainbow flags at community events and holding hands with their same-sex partners downtown. What Kerrie wasn't sure of, was how many other trans kids were in her community; she worried other parents would judge her, she didn't want to stand out, she wasn't ready to discuss medical interventions with anyone, and she just wanted to sit in the back of the room and listen.

When Kerrie arrived at the workshop, the tables were set up in a horseshoe shape – no back row to hide on. She almost left the class before it even started but lost her chance to flee discretely when the group leader began to speak. The leader introduced herself, shared her pronouns, and asked group members to do the same. The lady who went first was wearing a t-shirt that said "Proud Parent" over the background of a rainbow flag waving in the wind. She announced her name and her pronouns and rattled off a list of all her kids and their identities: "Sammy is our trans son, and Sarah thinks she's bi. . . ."

"Did she say, 'trans son'?" Kerrie thought.

In fact, she did! And, there were two other parents in the group whose children are trans. When it was Kerrie's turn to introduce herself to the group, she sat up straight and said, "Hi, I'm Kerrie. My son is trans, and I guess I'm just here to learn how to do the right things for him. That's all." When they'd gone all the way around the horseshoe, the group leader thanked everyone for sharing and directed participants to their workbooks.

As she worked through the exercises in Chapter 1 with the group, Kerrie realized she had just introduced Dani as her *son* for the first time, and she felt good about it. When she looked back at her work later in the week, Kerrie felt glad she committed to setting aside time for herself to engage with other parents, to learn new and changing things about herself, and to invest in being the best mom she can be to her son. Kerrie remembered claiming the right to "take time to adjust to a new-to-me reality" and, for the first time in weeks, didn't feel like she was falling behind or failing.

Reflection Questions

A moment to reflect.

At the end of each chapter, we will provide space for reflection. You may choose to answer the guided questions provided or use this space during the time between chapters to help you process your thoughts. It may be helpful to record milestones in your progress toward building a better relationship and providing an affirming home for your LGBTQ+ child (Egan et al., 2023). In short, use this space, however it best benefits you and your journey.

- What activity in this chapter was most challenging for you to complete? Why?
- Did you have a light bulb moment? How would you describe that moment to a friend?
- What are you looking forward to in the next chapter?
- What is one way you can show yourself compassion over the next week?

References

Abreu, R. L., Gonzalez, K. A., Rosario, C. C., Pulice-Farrow, L., & Rodríguez, M. M. D. (2020). "Latinos have a stronger attachment to the family": Latinx fathers' acceptance of their sexual minority children. *Journal of GLBT Family Studies, 16*(2), 192–210. https://doi.org/10.1080/1550428X.2019.1672232

Abreu, R. L., Martin, J. A., & Badio, K. S. (2023). Latinx LGBTQ people and their families: The role of Latinx cultural values, beliefs, and traditions. In J. M. Koch, E. E. Townsend-Bell, & R. D. Hubach (Eds.), *Identity as resilience in minoritized communities: Strengths-based approaches to research and practice* (pp. 47–58). Springer Nature Switzerland. https://doi.org/10.1007/978-3-031-38977-1_4

Austin, A., Craig, S. L., Matrese, M., Greeno, E., Weeks, A., & Bestinger, S. A. (2021). Preliminary effectiveness of an LGBTQ+ affirmative parenting intervention with foster parents. *Children and Youth Services Review, 127*. https://doi.org/10.1016/j.childyouth.2021.106107

Balmores-Paulino, R. S. (2020). Avoidance coping strategies. In V. Zeigler-Hill, & T. K. Shackelford (Eds.), *Encyclopedia of personality and individual differences* (pp. 343–344). Springer International Publishing.

D'amico, E., Julien, D., Tremblay, N., & Chartrand, E. (2015). Gay, lesbian, and bisexual youths coming out to their parents: Parental reactions and youths' outcomes. *Journal of GLBT Family Studies, 11*(5), 411–437. https://doi.org/10.1080/1550428X.2014.981627

Egan, J. D., Tolman, S., McBrayer, J. S., & Ballesteros, E. (2023). Reconceptualizing Kolb's learning cycle as episodic & lifelong. *Experiential Learning and Teaching in Higher Education, 6*(1), 24–33. https://doi.org/10.46787/elthe.v6i1.3607

Egolf, A., & Gold, A. L. (2023). Interpersonal effectiveness in action: The therapeutic milieu for DBT assertiveness skills practice. *Brown University Child & Adolescent Behavior Letter, 39*(3), 1–4. https://doi.org/10.1002/cbl.30693

Epton, T., Currie, S., & Armitage, C. J. (2017). Unique effects of setting goals on behavior change: Systematic review and meta-analysis. *Journal of Consulting and Clinical Psychology, 85*(12), 1182–1198. https://doi.org/10.1037/ccp0000260

Hawkins, J. D., Smith, B. H., & Catalano, R. F. (2004). Social development and social and emotional learning. In J. E. Zins, R. P. Weissberg, M. C. Wang, & H. J. Walberg (Eds.), *Building academic success on social and emotional learning: What does the research say?* (pp. 135–150). Teachers College Press.

Jefferson, F. A., Shires, A., & McAloon, J. (2020). Parenting self-compassion: A systematic review and meta-analysis. *Mindfulness*, *11*(9), 2067–2088. https://doi.org/10.1007/s12671-020-01401-x

Kayman, D. J., Goldstein, M. F., Dixon, L., & Goodman, M. (2015). Perspectives of suicidal veterans on safety planning. *Crisis*, *36*(5), 371–383. https://doi.org/10.1027/0227-5910/a000348

Lannin, D. G., Vogel, D. L., Guyll, M., & Seidman, A. J. (2019). Reducing threat responses to help-seeking information: Influences of self-affirmations and reassuring information. *Journal of Counseling Psychology*, *66*(3), 375–383. https://doi.org/10.1037/cou0000313

Morgan, H., Wells, L., Lin, A., Strauss, P., & Perry, Y. (2023). Parental challenges, facilitators and needs associated with supporting and accepting their trans child's gender. *LGBTQ+ Family: An Interdisciplinary Journal*, *19*(1), 70–86. https://doi.org/10.1080/27703371.2022.2142717

Rogers, M. L., Gai, A. R., Lieberman, A., Musacchio Schafer, K., & Joiner, T. E. (2022). Why does safety planning prevent suicidal behavior? *Professional Psychology: Research and Practice*, *53*(1), 33–41. https://doi.org/10.1037/pro0000427

Ryan, C., & Chen-Hayes, S. F. (2013). Educating and empowering families of lesbian, gay, bisexual, transgender, and questioning students. In E. S. Fisher, & K. Komosa-Hawkins (Eds.), *Creating safe and supportive learning environments* (pp. 209–229). Routledge.

Saenz, A. (2015). *Relationships that work: Four ways to connect (and set boundaries) with colleagues, students, and parents*. Routledge.

Testa, R. J., Habarth, J., Peta, J., Balsam, K., & Bockting, W. (2015). Development of the gender minority stress and resilience measure. *Psychology of Sexual Orientation and Gender Diversity*, *2*(1), 65–77. https://doi.org/10.1037/sgd0000081

Urmanche, A. A., Oliveira, J. T., Gonçalves, M. M., Eubanks, C. F., & Muran, J. C. (2019). Ambivalence, resistance, and alliance ruptures in psychotherapy: It's complicated. *Psychoanalytic Psychology*, *36*(2), 139–147. https://doi.org/10.1037/pap0000237

van Bergen, D. D., Wilson, B. D. M., Russell, S. T., Gordon, A. G., & Rothblum, E. D. (2021). Parental responses to coming out by lesbian, gay, bisexual, queer, pansexual, or two-spirited people across three age cohorts. *Journal of Marriage and Family*, *83*(4), 1116–1133. https://doi.org/10.1111/jomf.12731

Wilson, K. G., & Murrell, A. R. (2011). Values work in acceptance and commitment therapy. In S. C. Hayes, V. M. Follette, & M. M. Linehan (Eds.), *Mindfulness and acceptance: Expanding the cognitive-behavioral tradition*. Guilford Press.

CHAPTER 2

TERMINOLOGY AND FACTS YOUR QUEER KID (LIKELY) WANTS YOU TO KNOW

Language Matters

You might have heard the saying, "The only thing that never changes is that everything changes." In other words, the world is in a constant state of change. The beaten path we always used to take suddenly becomes a marshland and we have to find another path to our destination (or we splash through the water and deal with muddy, wet shoes). It is uncomfortable to find another path. In fact, it is a huge inconvenience, but it is part of life.

Language is another thing that constantly changes. English is a living language. That means we are always creating new words, using established words in different ways, and reorganizing the way we use words. This is definitely true when it comes to the ways we talk about people (Rossi & Lopez, 2017).

We would love to provide you with a list of words that describe LGBTQ+ teens that you could memorize. We wish you could carry around a pocket dictionary to pull out and look up the meaning of words your teen uses to describe themself or others. The uncomfortable truth, however, is that, as teens continue to explore their identities, they keep coming up with words to better describe those identities; a word that worked last year, may not work right now (Lawlis, 2022).

For example, when you were growing up, you might have heard the word "queer" used as an insult. Right now, lots of teens use "queer" to describe themselves, but that may not always be the case. We would be doing you a disservice if we gave you a list of words or identities to memorize. You might walk up to your teen and confidently call them "queer" only to discover that you made a big mistake.

In this chapter, we use current terms and we discuss common identities, but we encourage you not to get too caught up in the differences between, for example, "polyamorous" and "bisexual." Instead, we try to give you the tools to critically think about how identities are shaped, why terminology changes, and what it takes to affirm teens when they may not have all of the answers. We want to empower you to journey with them, when they are in the middle of figuring themselves out.

We are not saying that words don't matter because they ultimately change, rather, words matter very much and that is why they change (Rossi & Lopez, 2017). As humans, we are always searching for better and better words to describe our experiences. We are always in search of just the right word or concept to capture our experience.

We recommend a "wise knowing" approach to language (Salgado et al., 2019). A person who uses "wise knowing" is invested enough to figure out the current meaning of key words that describe LGBTQ+ experiences, but they are wise enough to flex and change their vocabulary along the way (Grossmann et al., 2024). For example, you might know that bisexual once applied to people who were attracted to men and women. Still, you are wise enough to accept when someone tells you they are bisexual, but that means they are attracted to people of multiple different genders.

DOI: 10.4324/9781003678205-2

In our work, we have found that teens appreciate when adults, especially parents, approach them with knowledge and wisdom. They appreciate knowing that parents care enough to learn about identities, but they also appreciate the room to grow, redefine themselves, and explain what terms mean to them, in their unique contexts (Medico et al., 2020; Pullen Sansfaçon et al., 2020). In other words, it is more important for parents to show they are invested in better understanding their children, as opposed to coming across as if they have all of the answers. If you really think about it, who likes a know-it-all?

After we've explored current terminology, we will take a look at what we're bringing with us on our parenting journey and as we take a baggage inventory. It is scary to move beyond your comfort zone and then realize that you loaded your hiking pack (and yourself) down with unhelpful items. When we feel safe and grounded, we might be likely to throw chocolate bars, soda, and other non-nourishing stuff into our backpacks, but at the top of the mountain, a bottle of water quenches thirst much better than a can of soda. We will help you to take stock of what you carry with you so that you can set a healthy, efficient plan for completing this journey.

We will continue to challenge our initial packing list by exploring myths and facts about LGBTQ+ people. We want to challenge you to look objectively (or as objectively as possible) at the ideas and beliefs you already hold about the LGBTQ+ community and to consider your sources of information. You may notice yourself comparing thoughts and ideas to your own family's experiences and starting to question things that just do not fit.

This chapter will conclude with a look at how you can take an active role in developing trust with your teen. Over the course of any relationship, trust and openness may ebb and flow, and it's vital to the relationship that we find moments to intentionally engage in actions that help build, maintain, and even rebuild trust. Remember that our society is not built with LGBTQ+ people in mind and the realities of living in a society where one finds themself a minority may lead to a tedious relationship with trust (Guest & Weinstein, 2020; Wilkes & Wu, 2018). Therefore, it is essential that you work to build a safe space where your teen can learn to trust you and your commitment to affirming them as their true, authentic self.

Step 5: The Erasable Dictionary

As we noted in the introduction to this unit, language is constantly changing and LGBTQ+ terminology is no exception (Rossi & Lopez, 2017). Parents who combine wisdom with knowledge ("wise knowing") understand common LGBTQ+ terms, but leave the door open for those terms to change. The next worksheet helps you define the meaning of common terms, but we ask that you fill in the blanks with pencil as a reminder that those definitions can change or can be interpreted in different ways by different people.

> Keep your eraser handy: The only thing that never changes is that everything changes.

The fact that terminology is constantly changing can make it easy to dismiss or discredit specific terms. You might hear people say, "What is the big deal about pronouns?" Usually, a word or phrase is upsetting or affirming to an individual because it connects with something deeply important to that person – perhaps their faith or the way they see themselves (Campbell et al., 2017; Money, 2023). Take a moment to consider what words are important to you and then consider that the words in this exercise may connect with the core of who your child is and, for that reason, they are important.

One way to learn key terms is to try to define them. Please take a moment to define the terms on the next page (in pencil!) and follow the instructions to show how confident you are in your definition. Once you've completed this activity, please check your answers against the answer key at the back of the workbook and make any necessary corrections (you can also correct the definitions at the end of the workbook if you've found them to be outdated).

It may also be useful to talk about terms that are important to your child's individual identity or experiences. Please feel free to add terms that are important to your family and their definitions on the blank lines at the bottom of your Erasable Dictionary.

As you think and learn more about the terms discussed here, you may find yourself wondering more about your child's individual identity. We have found it helpful to simply ask a person how they identify when you are unsure. It would be okay, for example, to say to your teen: "Are they/them pronouns still a good fit for you?" Another way to "ask" a person to share their identity with you is to offer yours. You might introduce yourself to your teen's friends by saying something like, "Hi, my name is ________ and my pronouns are ________________." We have found that by offering our own pronouns when we meet new people, we signal to them that it's safe for them to tell us their pronouns.

> You can read more about pronouns in Appendix B in the Activity 5 Scientific Basis paragraph.

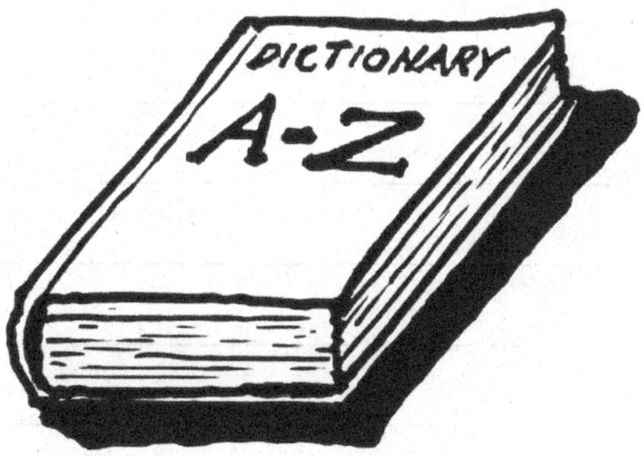

Image 2.1 The erasable dictionary.

Activity 5 My Erasable Dictionary

Please fill in the most current, accurate definition of the terms below. Then, indicate how sure you feel about the definition you wrote down by placing a number from 1 to 5 in the box. Higher numbers mean you are more sure and lower numbers mean you are less sure. The blank lines are provided so that you can add words that do not appear in the list already. If you want to check your answers against common definitions, check out the Activity 5 section in Appendix A.

☐ Asexual: ______

☐ Binary: ______

☐ Bisexual: ______

☐ Cis: ______

☐ Gay: ______

☐ Gender Expression: ______

☐ Gender Fluid: ______

☐ Gender Identity: ______

☐ Lesbian: ______

☐ Nonbinary: ______

☐ Pansexual: ______

☐ Queer: ______

☐ Questioning: ______

☐ Sexual Orientation: ______

☐ Trans: ______

☐ ______

☐ ______

☐ ______

☐ ______

Step 6: What I Carry With Me

As you filled out the erasable dictionary, you might have noticed yourself feeling frustrated, grumpy, or dismissive. We shared evidence that pronouns and identity terms matter, but if you have not had to question your identity over and over throughout your life, it can seem unnecessary. Your frustration and other emotions make sense and it is valid, but they can also be informative. In other words, your emotions can teach you a lot of things (Holodynski & Kärtner, 2023). In particular, grumpy emotions can teach you where you might be carrying baggage.

At this point in the journey, we'd like you to consider what "baggage" you carry with you that may inform your readiness, ability, and level of willingness to truly connect with and affirm your LGBTQ+ child. Baggage can be like water to a fish. You carry it so long (or swim around in water so long) that you stop noticing it. One way to start noticing baggage (or the water you swim in) is to start noticing your emotions (Rutherford, 2023). When you think about your child's identity, what makes you smile, laugh, cry, and want to yell?

Now that you are starting to "see the water" or notice your baggage, you are ready to do some even deeper thinking that takes you outside of your initial emotional responses. Take a moment to reflect on the values, beliefs, experiences, and assumptions you hold that may get in the way of fully benefiting from this workshop. You can jump ahead and start looking at the worksheet because these thoughts are going to factor into the activity.

As you think of pieces of baggage, you can go ahead and list them in under the "Baggage" heading in Activity 6, Baggage Inventory. Some examples of baggage might be: "I think all LGBTQ+ people are weird," or "I think I will lose all of my friends if they find out my kid is gay." Your baggage might more directly relate to your child such as: "I think my kid just wants to be special," or "This whole identity thing feels like a power play." One thing that makes baggage invisible is that it is plausible, defensible, or may even contain some truth, so just write your thoughts without trying to decide if they are true or not. You do not have to defend your baggage at this stage.

Now look back over your list of baggage and circle the things you want to bring with you. This should be only the baggage you are not ready to let go of. Notice that the exercise is not about dropping all of your baggage all at once.

We dig deeper into baggage in Appendix B Activity 6 Scientific Basis.

As we mentioned earlier in this workbook, it is important to be authentic and self-reflective during this journey (a common practice in Person-Centered Therapy; Rogers, 1951). Pretending something is not a big deal does not make it easier to deal with. In fact, ignoring what you care about can actually make things worse because you act out your feelings even when you ignore them.

Then, for each piece of baggage that you did not circle, write in an alternative, helpful item you would like to replace the baggage with under the "Tools" heading in Activity 6, Baggage Inventory. You will notice that you are not being asked to just drop the baggage you want to get rid of. Baggage can serve the purpose of supporting and grounding you. We want you to stay grounded and supported, so we are encouraging you to replace your supports, not drop and walk away from them.

For example, just like we suggested in the hiking metaphor that carrying water will be more helpful than soda, you could replace "I think all LGBTQ+ people are weird," with "My child is unique and I am committed to having a healthy, loving relationship with them." You could also keep the truth in your baggage, while replacing the unhelpful parts. For example, you could replace, "I think my kid just wants to be special," with "I can work on embracing my child for who they are so that they do not have to work so hard to get me to invest in them."

Lastly, consider actions you can take to turn baggage into tools. For example, if you're working on using the correct name or pronouns for your child, it might be helpful to update their contact in your cell phone address book. If you want to start spending more time showing your child they are special, you might need to change your schedule or actually put "time together" in your calendar. Working through your baggage takes intentional, action-orientated work.

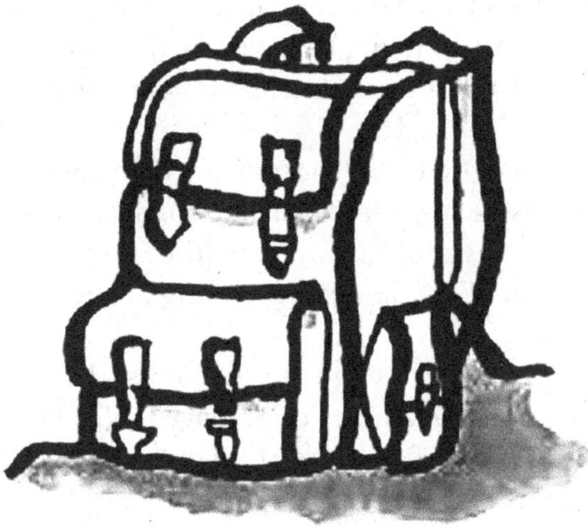

Image 2.2 Baggage and tools.

Activity 6 Baggage Inventory

Baggage	Tools

Action Items to Change Baggage into Tools

Step 7: Myths versus Facts

Another thing that makes baggage so hard to identify and challenge is the fact that it can also be connected to strong myths and misconceptions about LGBTQ+ people. There is a lot of misinformation out there (Garofalo, 2023). When teens come out to their parents, those myths can be triggered.

You can read more about core beliefs and triggers in the Appendix B Activity 7 Scientific Basis paragraph.

Parents can become tearful and say things like, "I just don't want you to die from AIDS," or "Does this mean you're doing drugs?"

If you are going to effectively replace and rework your baggage, you need to get familiar with key myths and misconceptions about LGBTQ+ youth. The next activity (Activity 7) will help you unpack some of the most common myths and facts about LGBTQ+ people. Go ahead and turn to that activity and follow the directions.

You can hop down to the activity and then come back to this spot when you are ready to reflect on the activity as a whole.

Now that you have had time to reflect on your answers and correct any misconceptions, please take time to answer the following questions. As you do, remember to reflect on your emotions and let them tell you something. For example, did you mark any statements as true that the workbook identified as false? Did you get all of the answers right? How do you feel as you reflect on your performance on this activity? Do your feelings of failure/success seem familiar when you think about parenting your LGBTQ+ child? Feel free to jot your thoughts below.

Misperceptions and myths come from somewhere. You did not spontaneously come up with your beliefs about LGBTQ+ people. You were most likely taught them (Bandura, 1977). Consider where you may have learned false information. What do you notice about those sources? Are there any notable commonalities or differences that, once identified, might help you to avoid false information in the future? Please jot your thoughts on the lines below.

Resistance can also be a sign of learning and deeply held beliefs (Lind & Thomsen, 2018). Just like it is important to learn from your emotions, it is also important to learn from your behaviors (Kolhe et al., 2024). If you notice yourself putting this workbook down or arguing with the answer key, you can learn from that too. Do you have any deeply felt disagreements with what the answer key identified as true? As false? What does that tell you?

____

____

Considering your answers above, what actions can you take to help yourself (and possibly others) reject false information about the LGBTQ+ community, especially when it is presented as fact? How can you continue wrestling with the answers that are hard to take in? How can you pick this book back up and recommit to journeying to the end?

____

____

Activity 7 True or False

Please circle the statements below that you think are true and X out the ones you think are false. After you have marked the statements as Myth or Fact, be sure to visit the answer key (in Appendix A under the Activity 7 section) at the back of this workbook and add a * or other symbol of your choosing to indicate which statements are actually factual. Try not to judge yourself for any answers you got wrong. These activities are not punitive; they are designed to help you grow. It may surprise you to know that even group leaders sometimes have to look up the answers!

LGBTQ+ people who get married do not stay together; the divorce rate is higher among LGBTQ+ couples.	The homelessness rate is higher among LGBTQ+ teens when compared to heterosexual, cis gender teens.	Nonbinary people are diagnosed with autism at high rates because being nonbinary messes people up.	Teens change their pronouns because it's a fad – it makes no difference in the long run what pronouns I use for my child.
Most people who transition from one gender to another (e.g. male to female) end up regretting that decision.	More LGBTQ+ teens identify as queer because it is popular, not because they really are LGBTQ+.	Being LGBTQ+ is a choice some humans make; it's not natural.	LGBTQ+ teens are more likely to get addicted to drugs and alcohol.
LGBTQ+ teens are at a higher risk for suicide due to rejection and discrimination.	It's not my place to correct someone if they use the wrong name or pronouns for my child.	Having just one affirming adult in their life can make a big difference in the mental health of an LGBTQ+ teen.	LGBTQ+ teens are highly resilient and able to counteract the impact of discrimination and oppression.
Being gay or lesbian is just about sex.	Polyamorous people just want to be promiscuous without any rules or standards.	Being LGBTQ+ is completely incompatible with being a person of faith.	I can have a strong relationship with my LGBTQ+ teen even though I do not accept their LGBTQ+ identity.

Step 8: Developing Trust

As you look over your teen's developmental history, you may see several places where trust between you and your child broke down. We believe that trust is an essential part of parenting, and it can be hard to maintain a consistent foundation of trust in a relationship with an LGBTQ+ teen (Mills-Koonce et al., 2018) that sometimes feels full of surprises (like the first time your teen came out to you). Take a moment to reflect on the first time your teen told you that they were LGBTQ+. Even if you were "totally cool with it," you might have felt sad that your teen took so long to tell you. You might have had thoughts like, "Why could they tell their sister, but not me?" or "Do they not trust me enough to share that part of their life?"

If you want to read more about the power of trust and relationship, you can turn to Appendix B and review the Activity 8 Scientific Basis Paragraph.

As you reflect, you may notice all sorts of ways your relationship with your teen can be impacted by ruptures or even breaches in trust. If those ruptures hurt you, it is probably safe to say that they also hurt your teen and during a person's teenage years, hormones, social media, social comparisons, and other influences can make typical hurts even more uncomfortable. Even the fear of a rupture can fill teens with fear. It may take them years of worrying before they share something big with you. However, the good news is that where breaches of trust have the power to hurt, deepening trust has the power to heal.

This is not a new concept. In Activity 4, we mentioned the concept of compound trauma or "death by a thousand bee stings." Traumatizing experiences are destabilizing, hurtful, and lead to disconnection (Campbell & Renshaw, 2018). One way to counteract the negative impact of trauma is to create community, relational stability, and trust (Schultz et al., 2016). We think of trust like a cup of refreshing water that gets you through a long hike. When you build trust, you have a full glass of cool water just when you need it. But when your cup has a hole in it (when your relationship with your teen breaks down over the years), you may raise it to your parched lips only to find it empty.

Trust involves sharing, but it is also important for parents and guardians to thoughtfully consider what to share and when. For example, it may feel good to share your anxieties about your paycheck and ability to pay bills, but does sharing that help your child? When deciding what to share with your teen, remember to consider developmental appropriateness (Meschke et al., 2012). Consider your teens age, their developmental age (which may or may not be the same as their chronological age), and the kinds of experiences they've had in their own life. Then ask yourself:

- How would what I share impact my teen at their current developmental stage? Am I sharing this to meet my needs or those of my teen?
- How will sharing this impact my relationship with my teen?
- If I share this, how can I keep my teen and myself safe?
- Can I still meet my need to share this information if I share it with someone other than my teen?

The following worksheet will help you strategize ways to restore and/or build trust, using the four ice cubes of connection. Just like ice cubes that melt and add cool refreshing water to your cup, these strategies will slowly refresh your relationship with your teen.

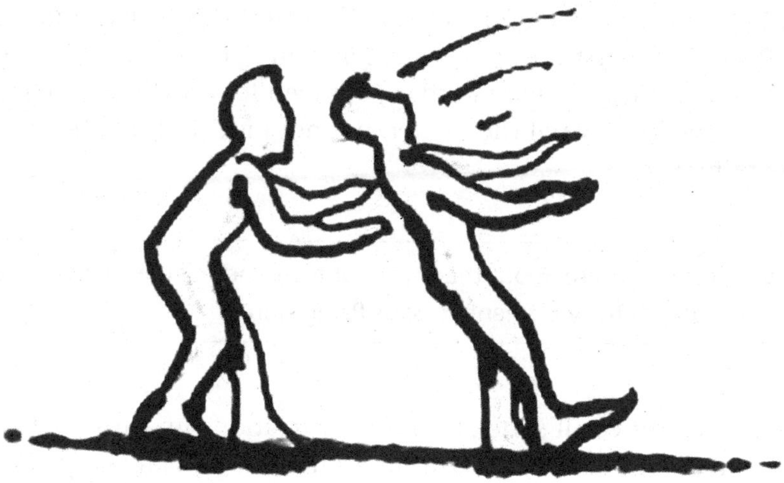

Image 2.3 The importance of trust.

Activity 8 Principles of Connection

One of the most effective ways to build trust and relationship with an LGBTQ+ person is simply by spending time with them. How could you work on spending more time with your teen?

Intimacy starts to take shape when we are intentional about the time we spend with someone. What kinds of activities can you do with your teen that might encourage deeper conversation? How can you show your teen that you're invested in learning more about them as they grow and develop into adulthood?

Another very effective way to build trust with an LGBTQ+ person is to love them for who they are. How could you work on doing more to celebrate your teen's unique personhood?

Your teen is more likely to share their life with you if you share yours with them. How could you work on sharing life with your teen to strengthen your relationship and help them feel safe to share theirs? Remember to keep it appropriate for your child's age and developmental level.

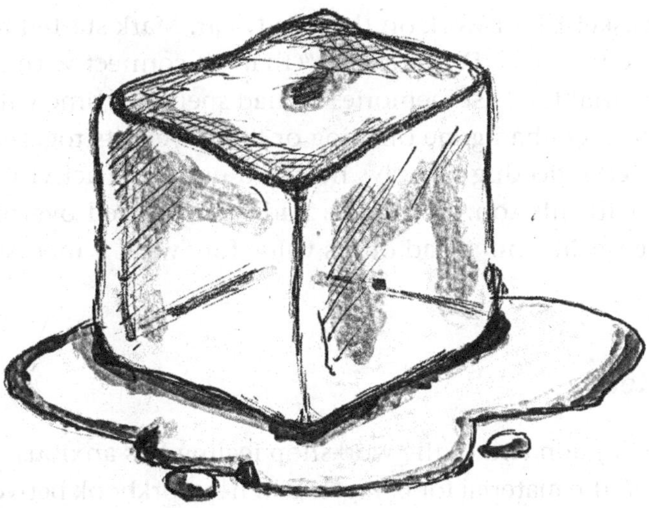

Image 2.4: Trust is refreshing.

Bringing It All Together

We covered a lot in this chapter. We asked you to dig into key concepts like identity and language, baggage, beliefs, and trust. The way you explore these themes in your own family may look different over time. In particular, trust-building is a complex process that can play out in unique ways in different families. We provide some examples here, but they are not exhaustive and should not serve as templates. They are just examples you can build on if that is helpful.

Vignette 3: Mark

Mark felt like the first chapter of the workbook was okay and he started noticing that it helped him connect with his son a little better. More than anything, it helped him to feel some empathy for Devin. He could still totally understand his wife's distress over Devin's disclosure, but Mark figured it would not hurt to keep "exploring things form Devin's point of view." Mark had always been curious and liked to try out new ideas even if he did not agree with them.

Engaging with the erasable dictionary and his exploration of his baggage helped Mark to realize how much the word "gay" called up images of AIDS, drug use, and images of "half-naked men parading down the street." It was almost therapeutic to erase that definition and write a new one.

The myth and fact activity helped Mark challenge his biases and zoom in on Devin's identity. At first, Mark had identified his son with the entire LGBTQ+ community. The myth and fact activity helped Mark realize that Devin had unique challenges and experiences as a gay man that might be related, but were somewhat different from other LGBTQ+ youth. Those insights helped Mark start thinking of his son as a person with common experiences as opposed to a stranger with weird behaviors and relationships.

After building more empathy and understanding, Mark felt ready to explore trust. For most of Devin's life, Mark had tried to build trust and connection with Devin by inviting Devin to play basketball or work on the family car. Mark started realizing he was more motivated by a desire to "make Devin a man" than to connect with his son. As he reflected, he started to notice that the best memories he had spending time with his son were drawn from times the two of them had gone on a jog or lifted weights together. After completing Chapter 2, Mark started reflecting on ways he could use those activities to build trust and shared understanding with his son. His values had not changed overnight, but he started trying to put his value for his son ahead of his value for "what a man should be like." He found it helped.

Vignette 4: Kerrie

Kerrie arrived at session two of the workshop feeling less anxious than she felt the first night. She had reviewed the material for Chapter 2 in her workbook between sessions, so she also felt prepared for what they would cover. When the leader started group, she reminded everyone that they are in a safe space for making mistakes and learning new concepts; this helped Kerrie feel even more at ease, especially because the language part of parenting an LGBTQ+ teen is something she found nerve-wracking.

The group worked through the Erasable Dictionary individually for several minutes and then the leader asked if there were terms that people struggled to define. Kerrie had struggled with a couple of the terms, but she felt fairly confident with many of them. She reflected on how much the language has changed since she was a teen and felt grateful that Dani had corrected her a few times and explained terms Kerrie didn't understand during conversation.

When the group moved on to work through the baggage activity, Kerrie was surprised to realize she was carrying baggage with her that she hadn't even noticed or connected to Dani's gender identity. Kerrie started to think back to the Identity Dream activity and how she had written down that one of her dreams for Dani was to be a mom . . . not a parent, not a dad, but a mom, specifically. All of the sudden Kerrie realized that, even though she felt accepting of Dani's gender identity, and even though she was gaining traction on adjusting the language she uses to talk about Dani (using his affirmed name and pronouns almost all the time, now), she hadn't yet fully realized just how much gendered language affects her ability to be affirming to her son. Then, she realized how intentional she will need to be as she works on becoming a more affirming parent to Dani.

The last activity in Chapter 2 was the one Kerrie was most excited about: She had noticed changes in her relationship with Dani over the last year or so and she wasn't totally sure if those changes were just normal teenage distancing or not. Whatever the cause, she thought this activity might help them begin to repair their relationship. Kerrie filled up the worksheet page with ideas about how to spend more time, be more intentional, share more of herself, and celebrate Dani's unique personhood. She decided to try at least two of her ideas out over the next week and see how Dani responds. She felt supported by the worksheet and the members of the group which, in turn, helped her to feel more confident about trying new methods of building trust and rebuilding her relationship with Dani.

Reflection Questions

Image 2.5 A moment to reflect.

- What activity in this chapter was most challenging for you to complete? Why?
- Did you have a lightbulb moment? How would you describe that moment to a friend?
- What are you looking forward to in the next chapter?
- What is one way you can work on building trust with your teen over the next week?

References

Bandura, A. (1977). *Social learning theory*. Prentice-Hall.

Campbell, S. B., & Renshaw, K. D. (2018). Posttraumatic stress disorder and relationship functioning: A comprehensive review and organizational framework. *Clinical Psychology Review*, *65*, 152–162. https://doi.org/10.1016/j.cpr.2018.08.003

Garofalo, R. (2023). Editor's Statement: Using misinformation to harm LGBTQ people is not new. *Transgender Health, 8*(4), 300–301. https://doi.org/10.1089/trgh.2023.29001.editorial

Grossmann, I., Peetz, J., Dorfman, A., Rotella, A., & Buehler, R. (2024). The wise mind balances the abstract and the concrete. *Open Mind: Discoveries in Cognitive Science, 8*, 826–858. https://doi.org/10.1162/opmi_a_00149

Guest, L. M. H., & Weinstein, N. (2020). The effect of healthcare provider support and discrimination on LGBT patients' trust and adherence. *The British Student Doctor Journal, 4*(3), 37–39. https://doi.org/10.18573/bsdj.204

Holodynski, M., & Kärtner, J. (2023). Parental coregulation of child emotions. In I. Roskam, J. J. Gross, & M. Mikolajczak (Eds.), *Emotion regulation and parenting* (pp. 129–148). Cambridge University Press.

Kolhe, C. S., Shikalgar, S., & Biggerstaff, D. (2024). Parental identity and lived experiences when parenting a LGBTQIA+2 child: A critical narrative synthesis of current evidence. *International Journal of Qualitative Studies on Health & Well-Being, 19*(1), 2738511. https://doi.org/10.1080/17482631.2024.2378511

Lawlis, S. M. (2022, January 7). Changing terminology in LGBTQ+ spaces: How to keep up with the lingo. *The Hospitalist.* https://blogs.the-hospitalist.org/content/changing-terminology-lgbtq-spaces-how-keep-lingo

Lind, M., & Thomsen, D. K. (2018). Functions of personal and vicarious life stories: Identity and empathy. *Memory, 26*(5), 672–682. https://doi.org/10.1080/09658211.2017.1395054

Medico, D., Pullen Sansfaçon, A., Zufferey, A., Galantino, G., Bosom, M., & Suerich-Gulick, F. (2020). Pathways to gender affirmation in trans youth: A qualitative and participative study with youth and their parents. *Clinical Child Psychology and Psychiatry, 25*(4), 1002–1014. https://doi.org/10.1177/1359104520938427

Meschke, L. L., Peter, C. R., & Bartholomae, S. (2012). Developmentally appropriate practice to promote healthy adolescent development: Integrating research and practice. *Child & Youth Care Forum, 41*(1), 89–108. https://doi.org/10.1007/s10566-011-9153-7

Mills-Koonce, W. R., Rehder, P. D., & McCurdy, A. L. (2018). The significance of parenting and parent–child relationships for sexual and gender minority adolescents. *Journal of Research on Adolescence, 28*(3), 637–649. https://doi.org/10.1111/jora.12404

Money, L. (2023). Labels and the self: Identity labels as scaffold. *Journal of Analytical Psychology, 68*(3), 590–609. https://doi.org/10.1111/1468-5922.12922

Pullen Sansfaçon, A., Medico, D., Suerich-Gulick, F., & Temple Newhook, J. (2020). "I knew that I wasn't cis, I knew that, but I didn't know exactly": Gender identity development, expression and affirmation in youth who access gender affirming medical care. *International Journal of Transgender Health, 21*(3), 307–320. https://doi.org/10.1080/26895269.2020.1756551

Rogers, C. R. (1951). *Client-centered therapy; its current practice, implications, and theory.* Houghton Mifflin.

Rossi, A. L., & Lopez, E. J. (2017). Contextualizing competence: Language and LGBT-based competency in health care. *Journal of Homosexuality, 64*(10), 1330–1349. https://doi.org/10.1080/00918369.2017.1321361

Rutherford, H. J. V. (2023). Neurobiology of parenting and implications for emotion regulation. In I. Roskam, J. J. Gross, & M. Mikolajczak (Eds.), *Emotion regulation and parenting* (pp. 229–243). Cambridge University Press.

Salgado, D. M., White, A. W., Peterson, D., & Dimeff, L. A. (2019). Cultivating wise mind in dialectical behavior therapy through mindfulness. In I. Ivtzan (Ed.), *Handbook of mindfulness-based programmes.* Routledge.

Schultz, K., Cattaneo, L. B., Sabina, C., Brunner, L., Jackson, S., & Serrata, J. V. (2016). Key roles of community connectedness in healing from trauma. *Psychology of Violence, 6*(1), 42–48. https://doi.org/10.1037/vio0000025

Wilkes, R., & Wu, C. (2018). Trust and minority groups. In E. M. Uslaner (Ed.), *The oxford handbook of social and political trust* (pp. 231–250). Oxford University Press.

CHAPTER 3

EVERYONE HAS AN IDENTITY JOURNEY . . . WHAT'S YOURS?

Looking Inward

At this point in our journey together, you may feel eager to jump ahead to more information about your teen. You might be wondering why it is important to look at yourself in a workshop that is focused on your child or children. Based on our experience and ongoing work with parents and guardians, we believe one of the best ways to figure out your teen, is to figure yourself out first. In other words, the better you understand yourself, the stronger the foundation you will have as you start working to better your relationship with your teenager (Post, 2025).

Self-understanding also builds empathy (Lind & Thomsen, 2018; Thomsen & Pillemer, 2017). It is easier to support and engage with your teen if you understand where they are coming from. LGBTQ+ teens may seem fundamentally different, but they are just people with typical problems, needs, and strengths (Vaughan & Rodriguez, 2014). As you explore your own needs, experiences, and identities, we invite you to think about how those parts of yourself give you a better understanding of your teen.

Looking inward may seem easy on the surface. You have lived your entire life with yourself. There is probably nobody else in this world you know better than you. But take a moment to reflect on some basic questions:

- When did you discover your gender?
- When did you realize that you were attracted to other people (or that you did not experience feelings of attraction like those around you)?
- What is your earliest memory of being your gender?

Questions like the ones above may come across as silly. Answers may just pop into your mind like, "I just knew," or, "This is how people like me are supposed to feel." If you are feeling frustrated or annoyed, please reflect on those feelings. They might help you understand why your LGBTQ+ teen gets frustrated when their gender or sexual orientation, something they have always felt or just know in the core of their being, is questioned. Questions about your identities may produce something as mild as an eye roll, but questions aimed at your teen about their identity can feel like a challenge, indictment, accusation, or disbelief.

As you work through this module, remember that taking an honest look at where you are in your journey to accepting and affirming your LGBTQ+ teen can stir up big feelings. Learning and growing in any area can be uncomfortable at times, like the fatigue that starts to set in as the incline of the trail steepens. It's okay to take a break when needed and to refer to your safety plan in Module 1 if you find yourself in need of extra support. This workbook is designed to bring you closer to your teen and we applaud you for doing the hard work necessary to affirm and support your child. At times like this, it

DOI: 10.4324/9781003678205-3

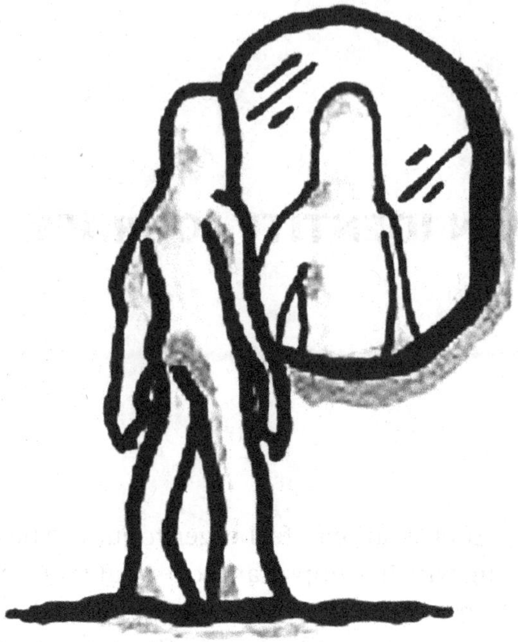

Image 3.1 An inward look.

is important to remember that, while what you are doing may be difficult, it is also incredibly valuable work.

We encourage you to take this module at your own pace. Please do not feel pressured to push yourself too far outside of your comfort zone. In psychology, there is something called a "vulnerability hangover" (Brown, 2012). When people share too much or push themselves too hard in a therapy session, they can feel regret and fear that what they said can't be taken back. Similarly, when people push themselves at the gym or on a hike, they can feel physically sore the next day. That soreness tells them that they taxed their muscles and opened themselves up for more growth. This feeling of soreness is much different than the pain that results when you tear a muscle from overexertion.

Sometimes work like this can produce a vulnerability hangover or a sense of worry or fear about oversharing or digging too deep. We have noticed in our own work that people often experience vulnerability hangovers after an impactful therapy session. We hope that the work you do in this unit will give you a mild sense of vulnerability that comes with growth or, in other words, "muscle soreness." We hope you will walk away feeling like you stretched yourself and now you can grow. We do not want you to experience a disruptive or long-term vulnerability hangover or (in terms of our exercise example), a "torn muscle." We do not want you to walk away feeling fearful, regretful, angry, or like it will take you a long time to bounce back. Only you can decide when your emotional muscles are overstressed, but the ideal approach is to stay in that optimal space of manageable discomfort.

Put simply, please take care of yourself as you work through this unit. It may help to remember that you are in a brave and supportive space with other parents who are doing the same work. You have control over your own sharing. The progress you make here is a gift to you that you can keep to yourself, only sharing it when you are ready.

Step 9: Identity as a Galaxy

Part of the reason terminology changes a lot is because people are on a constant journey of developing and finding themselves (Campbell et al., 2017). Because society is not set up to accept or affirm them,

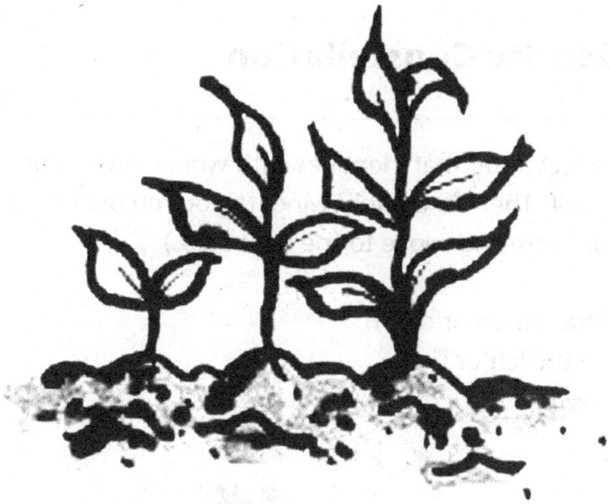

Image 3.2 Growth potential.

LGBTQ+ teens tend to really focus on their genders and sexual orientations, so they make new discoveries about themselves all the time. Even parents are on identity journeys full of discovery (Kolhe et al., 2024). This journey toward self-discovery is sometimes described as a journey through a galaxy.

If you want to read more about gender identity as multi-dimensional, you can turn to Appendix B the Activity 9 Scientific Basis paragraph.

Take a look at the galaxy in Activity 9 and think about how many stars fill a galaxy. There are millions! Now imagine that each of those stars is a unique identity. That is hard to do, isn't it? Humans like to make things simpler, so we tend to cluster or combine things that have similar characteristics or attributes. For example, you might be sitting in a chair as you read this book. There are probably other chairs in your house that look entirely different from the one you are sitting in, but most things designed to sit on, that have a flat spot (or seat) and are suspended above the ground in some way (e.g., with legs, attached to a wall, and so on) are called chairs. It is easier to get through life every day if you do not have to call every variety of chair something different and at the end of the day, chairs do not care what they are called.

Chairs do not get hurt if we make wrong assumptions about them or refer to them incorrectly. Humans are different. Sometimes when we group humans in clusters or based on characteristics we believe are most important, we miss the point and even create distress. In this activity, you get a chance to explore how somewhat small nuances make a big difference (even for you). You need some parameters, but you also need the freedom to explore. That's why we added four quadrants to the galaxy in this activity, to make it easy to navigate.

Activity 9 The Identity Constellation

For this exercise, please select a star that identifies with where you're comfortable and place the tip of your writing instrument on it. Then do the following: (If you run out of stars in any given direction, just stop at the edge of the universe and move to the next step.)

- Step 1: Move 3 stars straight up or down.
- Step 2: Move 7 stars to the left or right.
- Step 3: Move 4 stars up or down.

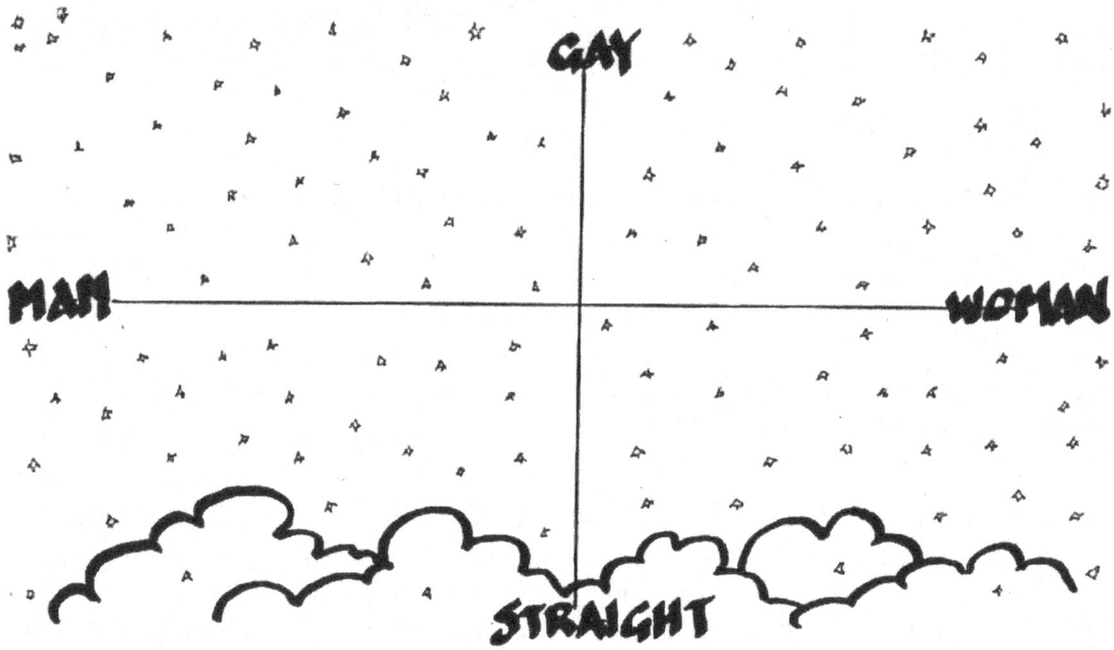

Image 3.3 A galaxy of identities to explore.

Now, imagine that the star you landed on and its corresponding quadrant are meant to reflect your gender identity/sexual orientation. Holding that "randomly assigned" identity in your mind, reflect on your thoughts and feelings by responding to the prompts that follow.

Try to imagine that everyone in your life sees and responds to you as the randomly assigned identity you landed on and write your reflections below.

How does it feel to be told that you have to be the identity you were assigned?

What changes or plans would you have to make if you were forced to stick with your new, randomly assigned identity? (For example, where would you no longer be able to go? What bathroom would you have to use? What sports could you play/not play?)

How do you see this experience as similar or different to your teen's experiences in relation to their unique identity as an LGBTQ+ person?

Step 10: My Unique Identities

In the previous exercise, we talked about the fact that gender and sexual orientation development is not linear. People may take two steps forward and one step back in their developmental process. They may skip steps or get stuck. For example, some people come out very early in their lives, whereas some people do not connect the dots and/or verbalize their identities until well into adulthood. Other people come out in stages. We will talk about coming out later in this workbook, but we use these examples to show how different each person's journey can be.

In the next exercise, we will ask you to reflect on your "current" identities. That is because our experiences of our sexual orientation and gender identity can change over time (Lindley et al., 2021). Please take a moment to think back to the last chapter in which you challenged your biases that being LGBTQ+ is a choice. There is a difference between recognizing that identity changes over time and suggesting that people choose their LGBTQ+ identities. The emphasis here is on discovery.

Because society tends to reject LGBTQ+ people or is at least set up to privilege people who are not LGBTQ+, people may lack the words to describe themselves. We have heard LGBTQ+ people talk about seeing the word "homosexual" in a dictionary for the first time and suddenly realizing that word describes them. Our world works through words, and if you do not have the word or concept to describe yourself, it can be hard to build self-understanding (see Knutson et al., 2024).

In the next activity, we are going to ask you to locate your current identity on a line.

> Curious about the rationale behind this section? You can read more about the importance of self-understanding in the Appendix B Activity 10 Scientific Basis section.

You might be wondering, "After you told me identity is a galaxy, why are you using lines and binaries?" We designed this exercise because, regardless of how aware of identity development you may become, society will still try to force you and your teen into predetermined categories. Thinking through those categories can be a source of growth. Please pay attention to any feelings you experience as you follow the directions. Paying attention to your thoughts and feelings can help you build empathy with your teen. It can point out differences and similarities that may impact their relationship with you.

Activity 10 How I Identify

Try filling out the diagrams below as thoughtfully and accurately as possible by placing the tip of your pen in the center of the line and sliding it to the location that best represents you. Place an X there.

A. My Current Gender Identity:

Man--Woman

☐ Nonbinary

B. My Current Gender Expression:

Masculine------------------------------------Androgynous--Feminine

☐ Nonbinary

C. My Current Sexual Orientation:

Gay/Lesbian--------------------------------------Bisexual-------------------------------------Heterosexual

☐ Asexual

Or Self-Identify

If the activity above frustrated you or if you did not feel you fit on one or more of the lines above, feel free to place your X's here _____. It is okay to self-identify outside of the options you were provided. It is possible that your teen does too. In fact, you can revisit this activity throughout your life to identify any changes in the ways you experience your gender and sexual orientation. Just like you, your teen's understanding of their identities may change and develop as they learn and grow.

D. My Gender Expression Over Time:

On the graph below, please chart your gender expression over time. For people who have had a relatively stable gender expression, their graph might look like a straight line, horizontal to the X axis. For people with gender expressions that have changed, their graph may look like the peaks and valleys of a mountainous hike. Please challenge yourself to be as accurate as possible – even the straightest path may fluctuate over time.

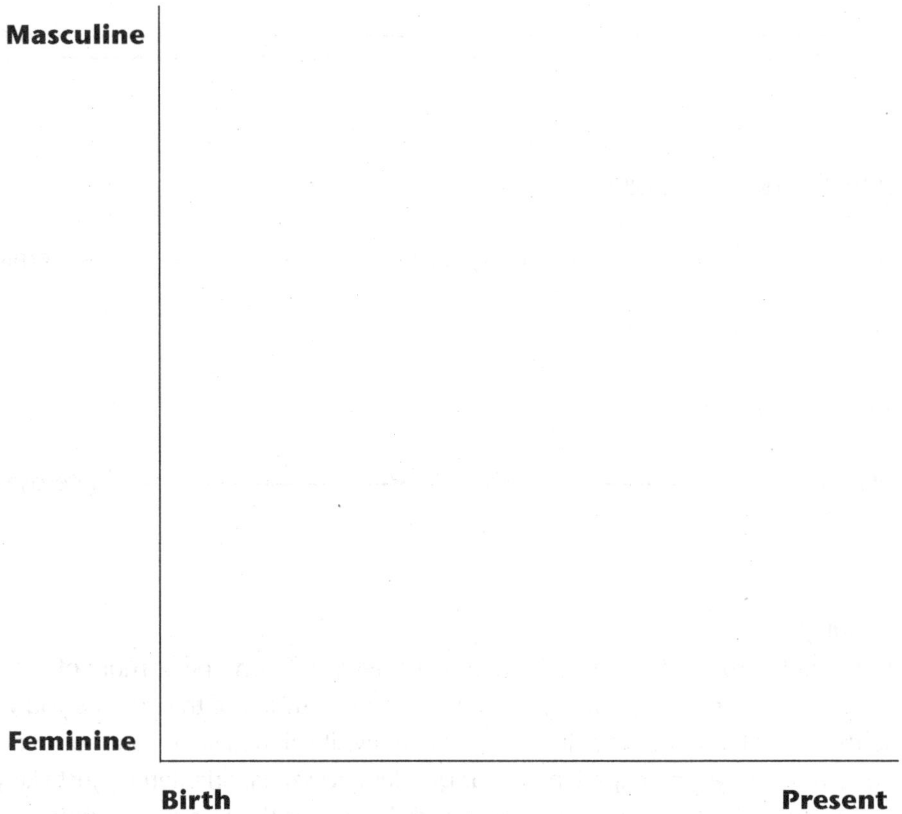

E. Deeper Reflection

If you want to dig deeper into this activity, you can reflect on the following questions:

- Do you feel comforted by the linear, binary design of the activity?
- Do you feel frustrated and want to skip the activity because it just feels wrong?
- How do you imagine your teen would feel about the activity?
- How long did it take you to notice that you could opt out by placing your "X" in the self-identify section?
- How did it feel to self-identify (if you ended up doing so)?

Step 11: Identity Penalties

If you have ever stepped outside of people's expectations for you (based on your gender or sexual orientation), you have probably been corrected or penalized in some way. For example, if you identify as a man and you cry, people may make fun of you or call you a wuss. If you identify as a woman and you join the military, you may be jokingly called a tomboy. There are small and big ways that we get corrected when we step out of line, especially when it comes to social expectations of our gender and sexual orientation (Walker, 2018). That happens to our teens as well.

> For more information about this exercise, see the Appendix B Activity 12 Scientific Basis paragraph.

As you prepare to engage with the next worksheet, please take a moment to think back to our hiking metaphor. When you are on the trail, you are safe and behaving like everyone expects. When you venture off the trail, however, you may be in danger of getting lost, bitten by a snake, or worse. At most state parks, park rangers take steps to keep people safe on challenging trails. They put out warning signs, add guardrails, and patrol different areas. In a similar way, people in society (and society itself) can work very hard to keep people from deviating too far from the beaten path of societal expectations.

Penalties for deviating from gender norms can range from snide comments, bullying, and even violence (González-González et al., 2025). Our use of the trail metaphor is not intended to trivialize the very real risks of deviating from societal expectations. However, the core idea is the same: Staying on the path is typically safe and leaving it can be very dangerous. Even snide comments or hurtful words, said over and over, can have a very painful combined effect. We discuss that combined or compound effect more in later chapters.

Take 5 minutes to think about your own thoughts, feelings, and behaviors as they relate to social expectations for your gender and/or sexual orientation. For most people, some of your thoughts, feelings, and behaviors will align or agree with social expectations for your gender or sexual orientation and other thoughts, feelings, and behaviors will not agree with what society expects of someone with your gender or sexual orientation identity. For example, if you identify as a man, you might have "acceptable" thoughts, behaviors, and feelings like:

- I like to work on cars.
- I enjoy watching football.
- I am attracted to women.

At the same time, you might notice thoughts, behaviors, and feelings that you are likely to get judged for:

- I like watching romantic comedies.
- I listen to queer artists.
- I am a "stay-at-home dad."

The important thing to remember is that none of these thoughts, feelings, and behaviors are "wrong." Living in society just makes some thoughts, feelings, and behaviors easier to embrace and share than others.

Activity 11 Walking the Path of Expectations

Using the following image, write the thoughts, feelings, or behaviors that society says align with your gender/sexual orientation identity inside the path. Then, write the thoughts, feelings, or behaviors that society says do not align with your gender/sexual orientation identity outside the path.

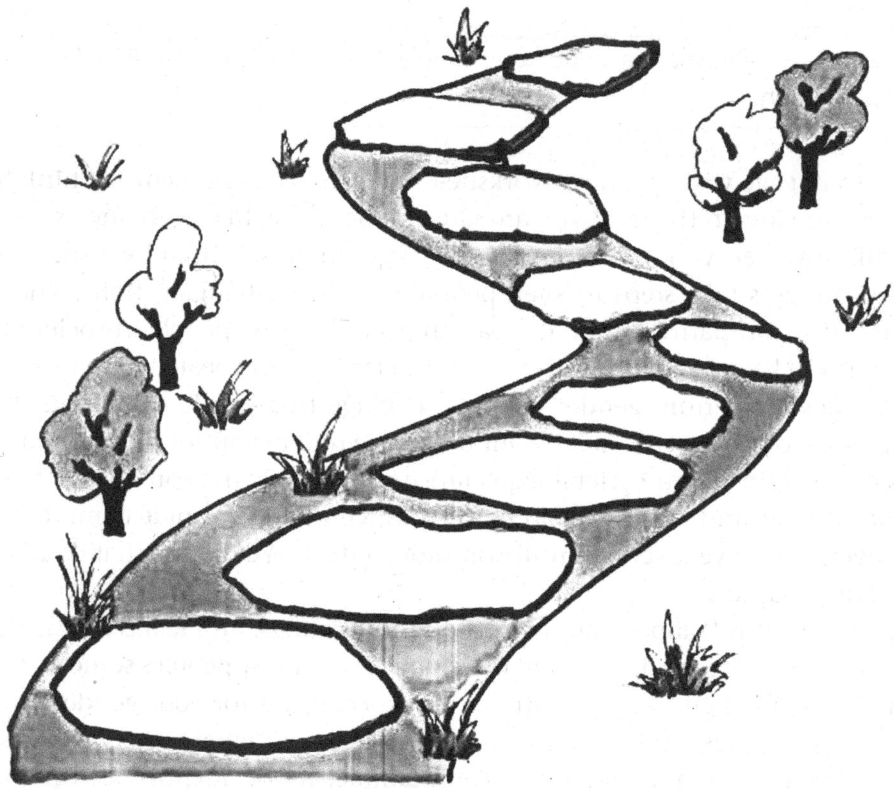

Image 3.4 The path of expectations.

Step 12: Working Through Emotions

We know these worksheets have probably been challenging to get through at times. You have been asked to reflect on the negative ways you have been treated when your thoughts, feelings, and behaviors have been rejected by others. You have also been asked to consider disappointment or unfulfilled dreams you may have had for your teen. That is tough work, but your willingness to stick with this process is also an accomplishment. We hope you will take a moment to reflect and acknowledge that you stayed with it and that is a valuable accomplishment.

The things you feel as you work through this workbook (disappointment, sadness, accomplishment, pride) are all powerful emotions. The thing about powerful emotions is that they can be hard to ignore and they often need to be shared. That is a hard need to meet if your feelings put you at risk of rejection, discrimination, or isolation. That is part of the reason we designed this workbook to be delivered in groups. In our experience, rural parents with LGBTQ+ youth rarely have someone to turn to when they need to share their fears, dreams, and experiences.

When you feel strong emotions about your teen, it can be hard not to share those emotions with them, especially if you do not feel like you are able to talk to other people such as family members, friends, or colleagues. However, your teen may not be ready to help you manage your emotions while they are managing their own emotions and experiences. They probably need someone to talk to themselves, and they may not have their own listening ear. What's more, releasing powerful emotions right away can actually backfire. They tend to come out in a disorganized, confusing jumble.

In other words, even if you have a hard time expressing your emotions or finding someone to listen, it can be very healing to sort those emotions out.

For more information about emotional expression, you can turn to the Appendix B Activity 12 Scientific Basis paragraph.

Sometimes, powerful emotions can be referred to as "secondary emotions." This means that they are the ones to show up and be noticed by others first, but they are actually based on a lot of other emotions that people are less likely to see. For example, when people get cornered, confused, or sad, they may express these primary emotions as anger. This worksheet gives you the opportunity to acknowledge and process tough emotions.

On the next page, you will find an emotional awareness building activity. Sigmund Freud used the metaphor of an iceberg to explain that people have emotions they are aware of (what shows above the water) and emotions they are unaware of (what is underneath the water), both of which are important (Scherer, 2005). As you know, icebergs are massive, but only a small part of the iceberg is visible above the water. Our emotions work in a similar way. We may feel a lot of things (below the surface of our consciousness), but we tend to focus on one major emotion when we are distressed (Scherer, 2005). In other words, the tip of the iceberg is what everyone tends to see (above the water), but the biggest part of the emotional experience happens behind the scenes (the part that is big enough to sink the Titanic).

Activity 12 Emotional Awareness

Please write the main emotion you feel when engaging with your LGBTQ+ teen about their identity at the top of the iceberg. It might be sadness, anger, confusion, or even joy or pride. This is the main emotion or the emotion that pops into your head right away. Next, break that emotion down by writing other emotion words below the water level. For example, if your major emotion is confusion, you might be feeling frustrated, anxious, isolated, lost, and so on (below the surface of the water). These are the supporting emotions (secondary to the main emotion) that you have to dig deeper to find.

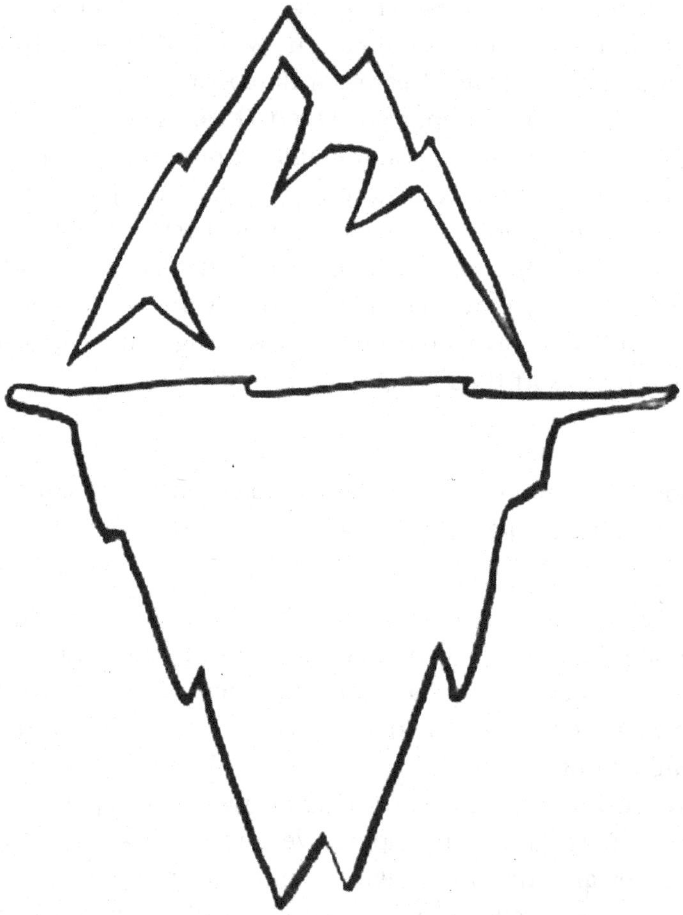

Image 3.5 Identifying emotions.

Bringing It All Together

As in previous chapters, you are encouraged to read over the following vignettes and reflect on how similar or different they are from your own experience. You can even write your own vignette if you want. Or you can share your thoughts and feelings with your group if you are completing the workbook with other people. This section is designed to help you tie the chapter together and reflect on what you have learned across all the activities in this chapter.

Vignette 5: Mark

Mark felt skeptical as he started reading over Chapter 3. He noticed references to feminist theory and gender exploration activities. It was hard for him to resist seeing the whole chapter as a bunch of gender theory ramblings. Mark's family got fiber internet a few years ago, but their rural location made it hard to get free T.V. channels and they had decided not to subscribe to streaming services. The family's primary source of information was YouTube. When not working on the farm, Mark would most often unwind watching conservative influencers, MMA reruns, or clips from conservative news stations.

Most of the influencers and news anchors Mark watched made disparaging comments about LGBTQ+ people. The YouTube clips tended to frame LGBTQ+ people as a threat to society and Mark's rural way of life. He was inclined to skip Chapter 3, but he ultimately decided "What the heck? Reading a book can't make me gay." The first two chapters seemed obvious, but the path exercise really got him thinking. He suddenly started to see how the YouTube videos he enjoyed watching were designed to "keep people on the path." In some ways, the influencers he watched seemed to be using LGBTQ+ people to market their videos and their arguments seemed kind of manipulative.

That caused Mark to reflect on ways he had been "kept on the path" himself. He noticed that there were ways he felt that he never shared because he was afraid people would think he was weak. As he completed the emotion iceberg, he noticed that he usually only expressed anger . . . because that was a safe emotion. He started to see why his son, Devin, had been so withdrawn and quiet lately. Mark's primary emotions for his son grew out of care and confusion, but he was most likely to express them as anger. It dawned on him that the care he was expressing was coming across as aggression and rejection. He decided to start exploring ways to express himself without "blowing up."

Vignette 6: Kerrie

When Kerrie arrived at group for the third week, she felt energized. She had stayed committed to working on building trust with Dani after session 2 and felt encouraged when Dani seemed to be more open with her. She had practiced using Dani's affirmed name and pronouns with close friends and changed his name in her phone contacts to read, "Dani, he/him."

As the group leader began the evening's discussion, Kerrie found herself clinging nervously to the title of the first section, "Looking Inward." Kerrie wasn't sure she had much to share – she *knew* she was a woman, and she *knew* she was attracted to men. She wondered why her experience would be important to understanding her son's, which was, as he had informed her more than once, a completely different story.

As she worked through the first activity, Kerrie found that she had landed on a star in the *Identity Constellation* that labeled her a gay man. She reflected on how she might feel if everyone else in her life saw her as a man and how frustrating that would be. She even remembered a particularly bad haircut she had gotten in the first grade that led to relentless teasing and other kids telling her she looked like a boy. She remembered how angry she felt when they would say that and how she committed to wearing dresses every day until her hair grew out and the teasing stopped.

Suddenly, Kerrie felt a lump in her throat. When the group reached the *Emotion Iceberg* activity at the end of Chapter 3, Kerrie realized she had experienced many emotions in the last 90 minutes since group began. She arrived feeling energized and excited about the progress she and Dani seemed to be making within their relationship, she felt sad and bothered when she relived her first grade haircut experience, she felt seen when she marked her current identities and mapped out her gender expression over time, and she felt angry when she reflected on the gender penalties she'd suffered for having short hair, enjoying fishing and mechanics over makeup and shopping, and when she was passed up for a promotion at work and a male colleague with less experience was promoted instead.

When Kerrie began to fill in the blanks on her emotion iceberg, she wrote the word "determined" at the top. She was determined to learn how to best support her son. As she filled in the secondary emotions, she realized that all the emotions she had experienced that night were fueling that determination and empowering her to continue the work she started when she signed up for this workshop. Feeling a little overwhelmed by everything that came up during group, Kerrie decided to take a drive before heading home. She listened to her favorite tunes on the stereo, savored a piece of "emergency chocolate" she kept in her purse for stressful days, and she took time to relax, breathe, and begin to process all the thoughts and ideas that were swirling through her mind.

Reflection Questions

Image 3.6 A moment to reflect.

- What activity in Module 3 was most challenging for you to complete? Why?
- Did you have a lightbulb moment? How would you describe that moment to a friend?
- What are you looking forward to in the next module?
- Over the next week, reflect on ways you might impose identity penalties or expectations on other people.

References

Brown, B. (2012). *Daring greatly: How the courage to be vulnerable transforms the way we live, love, parent, and lead.* Penguin Random House.

Campbell, D. G., Guimarães, J. A. C., Pinho, F. A., Martínez-Ávila, D., & Nascimento, F. A. (2017). The terminological polyhedron in LGBTQ terminology: Self-naming as a power to empower in knowledge organization. *Knowledge Organization, 44*(8), 586–591. https://doi.org/10.5771/0943-7444-2017-8-586

González-González, F., Strizzi, J. M., & Fernández-Agis, I. (2025). "Accepting a transgender child is to improve the way one lives on this planet": Support and acceptance trajectories of parents of transgender and gender diverse children. *LGBTQ+ Family: An Interdisciplinary Journal, 21*(2), 101–115. https://doi.org/10.1080/27703371.2024.2370883

Knutson, D., Goldbach, C., Kler, S., Rodriguez-Ordonez, I., Goff, B., & McDurmon, G. (2024). Language matters: Gender pronouns and identity terminology for transgender and nonbinary people. In J. A. Gedro, & T. S. Rocco (Eds.), *Routledge companion of LGBTQ identity in global, social, political, and work contexts*. Routledge. https://doi.org/10.4324/9781003128151

Kolhe, C. S., Shikalgar, S., & Biggerstaff, D. (2024). Parental identity and lived experiences when parenting a LGBTQIA+2 child: A critical narrative synthesis of current evidence. *International Journal of Qualitative Studies on Health & Well-Being*, *19*(1), 2738511. https://doi.org/10.1080/17482631.2024.2378511

Lind, M., & Thomsen, D. K. (2018). Functions of personal and vicarious life stories: Identity and empathy. *Memory*, *26*(5), 672–682. https://doi.org/10.1080/09658211.2017.1395054

Lindley, L. M., Nagoshi, J. L., Nagoshi, C. T., Hess III, R., & Boscia, A. (2021). An eco-developmental framework on the intersectionality of gender and sexual identities in transgender individuals. *Psychology & Sexuality*, *12*(3), 261–278. https://doi.org/10.1080/19419899.2020.1713873

Post, G. (2025). Resilient parents; resilient kids: How parental self-awareness is critical to helping smart kids thrive. *Gifted Education International*, *41*(1), 92–111. https://doi.org/10.1177/02614294241274442

Scherer, K. R. (2005). Unconscious processes in emotion: The bulk of the iceberg. In L. F. Barrett, P. M. Niedenthal, & P. Winkielman (Eds.), *Emotion and consciousness* (pp. 312–334). The Guilford Press.

Thomsen, D. K., & Pillemer, D. B. (2017). I know my story and i know your story: Developing a conceptual framework for vicarious life stories. *Journal of Personality*, *85*(4), 464–480. https://doi.org/10.1111/jopy.12253

Vaughan, M. D., & Rodriguez, E. M. (2014). LGBT strengths: Incorporating positive psychology into theory, research, training, and practice. *Psychology of Sexual Orientation and Gender Diversity*, *1*(4), 325–334. https://doi.org/10.1037/sgd0000053

Walker, A. (2018). *Collective consciousness and gender*. Palgrave Macmillan UK. https://doi.org/10.1057/978-1-137-54414-8

CHAPTER 4

GROWING UP LGBTQ+

The Basics

Development and Growth

As you journey through life with your LGBTQ+ teen, you may notice differences between your teen and other adolescents. For example, before the age of 7-years-old, boys and girls tend to play together in equally mixed groups. However, around age 7, boys and girls begin to segregate into same-gender play groups. In other words, boys play with boys and girls play with girls (Martin & Fabes, 2001).

However, you might notice that your LGBTQ+ teenage boy tends to spend most of his time with girls. Compared to the behavior of his peers, your teen's behavior may appear odd or unusual. In short, the way your teen grows and develops socially may be different from other teens in your life. United States societal norms enforce some pretty strict gender roles and expectations and when a teen deviates from those expectations it can be distressing for parents.

Worry and distress can cause a person to hyper focus or ruminate (think about something over and over) on a perceived source of distress (Willner, 1968). For a parent, it can be easy to become fixated on ways their teen deviates from societal expectations, picking apart all the little signs that their child might, or might not be LGBTQ+ for example. We would suggest that over-focusing on a teen's behaviors in an effort to determine their sexual orientation and/or gender identity is unhelpful and often leads to stereotypes. The reality is that there is no clear path from conception to LGBTQ+ identity. People express their genders in all sorts of ways (Pullen Sansfaçon et al., 2020) and that does not make them queer, it just makes them human.

What we mean is that sexual orientation and gender identity are influenced by complex interactions between genetics, physiology, and environment (Legato, 2020). In fact, there are natural variations in gender, biological sex, and sexual orientation across several species of animals, including humans (Roughgarden, 2013; Sommer & Vasey, 2006). Medical science tells us that while most people fall into the well-known binary categories of male and female sex, humans can be born with many combinations of chromosomes, anatomy, and hormones (Kennedy, 2024). What's more, gender norms change over time so that something that was once acceptable for men (e.g., wearing makeup, wigs, or skirts) becomes unacceptable later in history (Haines et al., 2016). This means there is nothing essentially or inherently gendered about clothes, shoes, accessories, makeup, or specific gestures, and their meaning and acceptability can change over time.

In the past, there have been attempts to change or "treat" LGBTQ+ identities through practices known as conversion therapy or reparative therapy. Through scientific research and clinical practice, we now know that these practices are harmful and ineffective (Cramer et al., 2008; Haldeman, 2022). Now, conversion therapy has been denounced or banned by major healthcare organizations, including the American Medical Association (2022), American Psychological Association (2009), and American Academy of Child & Adolescent Psychiatry (2018).

In some ways, this information might come as a relief: You did not make your teen LGBTQ+ by loving them too much, coddling them, traumatizing them, or through any other parenting choice you've made.

DOI: 10.4324/9781003678205-4

Rather, having an LGBTQ+ teen gives you the opportunity to succeed more as a parent than you ever could have imagined. In other ways, it can be hard to accept that your teen just happens to be LGBTQ+ because humans don't do well with ambiguity, and we want solid answers (Imaz-Sheinbaum, 2021).

In this workbook, we will ask you to embrace the ambiguity involved in parenting an LGBTQ+ teen. Just as you probably don't sit back and worry about how your heterosexual/cisgender children/nephews/nieces ended up the way they are, it usually doesn't add much to your skill as a parent to overly reflect on how your LGBTQ+ teen ended up the way they are. We want to recognize that you are engaging in a workbook focused on parenting LGBTQ+ teens, as if there is something fundamentally different or challenging about LGBTQ+ teens, but the reality is that they are pretty mundane and a lot like all other teens (Ceatha et al., 2021). The major difference is that LGBTQ+ people do not fit into society yet and the discrimination they feel can make typical teenage problems and experiences harder to get through (Tarantino & Jamison, 2023; Testa et al., 2015).

In other words, adolescence is a tumultuous time for all teens – the adolescent brain is restructuring itself to best handle current needs; social needs and expectations are changing (biologically speaking, finding a peer group is tied directly to survival); hormones are changing, and more (O'Donohue et al., 2013). LGBTQ+ teens experience all the same developmental changes as their heterosexual, cis peers, plus the additional struggles that result from identity-based rejection, isolation, or gender dysphoria (e.g., Hafeez et al., 2017).

Step 13: My Changes Throughout Adolescence

This chapter is designed to help you explore your LGBTQ+ teen's individual developmental process in a way that helps you better support and affirm your teen. Doing so helps you to avoid pitfalls such as unhelpful stereotypes, assumptions that your teen is just like other LGBTQ+ teens, and so on. By now, you should notice how each chapter builds on the next. You have already challenged broad stereotypes and explored your own identities. You will apply many of those foundational insights in this chapter. As usual, we will start with a focus on you.

During adolescence, teens dream big dreams, make ever changing plans for the future, and try out relationships with other teens (Newman & Newman, 2020). Before you focus on your teen's development, we encourage you to focus on your own adolescent years.

To read more about dynamics involved in focusing on development, you can turn to the Appendix B Activity 13 Scientific Basis paragraph.

As you reflect on your own experience, you may notice that a lot of things changed for you between when you were a teen and where you are in life now. In Chapter 3, we talked about the fact that "change" is different from "choice." Many of your interests change throughout your lifespan and many of those changes seem almost automatic or subconscious. Sometimes, those changes are influenced by friends, media, or your parents.

For example, you might have gotten fixated on a specific brand and refused to wear anything else. You might have had bangs or dreamed of being an artist. You might have written poetry or longed for a person whose name you can no longer remember. You will notice that none of those changes are bad, they are just changes. They all combined to make you the person you are today. The same is true for your teen. You are watching them develop (sometimes in very hard to detect ways) into the person they will be someday.

Activity 13 Changes Across the Lifespan

As you reflect, please fill out the table below in response to each prompt. Across from the prompt, please jot notes about the plans/expectations you had as an adolescent (my plans), the way things actually turned out (your current reality), and any thoughts about the difference between your early dreams and current reality (the outcomes). For example, maybe you planned to be a doctor, but you ended up becoming an accountant. Were you or others thrilled/disappointed about this outcome?

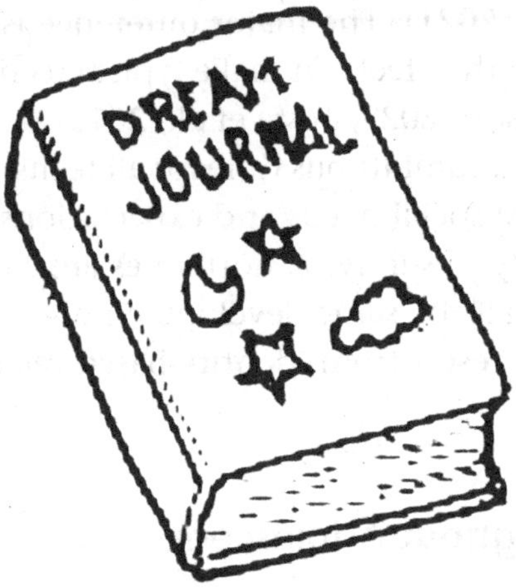

Image 4.1 Dreams for my future.

Prompt	My Plans/ Expectations	My Current Reality	The Outcomes/ Implications
What you wanted to be when you grew up.			
Who you wanted to marry/spend your life with.			
What you planned to do for work.			
Where you planned to live.			
How much money you planned to make.			
How many children you planned to have.			
Your best friend for life.			

Step 14: Myths and Facts of Adolescence

There are lots of rumors and misconceptions that circulate about LGBTQ+ adolescent development (Abreu et al., 2017; Newcomb et al., 2018). It can be hard to separate the myths from the facts. When parents and caregivers base their assumptions about their teens on myths, they often end up unnecessarily beating themselves up or examining their teen's behaviors for any clue about their LGBTQ+ identity.

We discuss the power of assumptions further in the Appendix B Activity 14 Scientific Basis paragraph.

That dynamic also works in reverse. Once a parent knows their teen is LGBTQ+, they may start blaming their teen's behaviors (usually misbehaviors) on their teen's identity. As we discussed in Chapter 3, there are lots of ways that people deviate from gendered expectations every day. Some of those behaviors get punished (with insults or jabs), but many go unnoticed. However, for LGBTQ+ youth, deviations from the norm tend to stick out more and get noticed more often. Those deviations can be unfairly linked to a teen's identity and even completely unrelated behaviors (e.g., skipping class, staying out late, trying marijuana) can get blamed on the fact that they are LGBTQ+. Among other things, the process of assuming that one aspect of a person's identity is responsible for everything you dislike about them is called stigmatization or stereotyping (Schneider, 2021).

This is an important place to again acknowledge that LGBTQ+ teens are like any other teen. They want to fit in, make silly mistakes, and are capable of amazing things. This activity is focused on breaking down stigma, demystifying LGBTQ+ identity, and demonstrating that even though growing up LGBTQ+ can carry with it a lot of challenges and opportunities, much of a teen's experience in adolescence (e.g., whether they make an "A" on a test or like spaghetti) has little to do with whether or not they are LGBTQ+.

The activity you are about to complete may feel familiar. You have already worked through general myths and facts about LGBTQ+ youth in Chapter 2. However, this exercise is a little different. This time, we want you to reflect on a bunch of statements about development so you can get practice separating common myths from key facts. Similar to the previous activity, please circle statements you think are true and put an "X" through statements you think are false.

Activity 14 Identifying Myths and Facts

After completing the activity, take a moment to reflect on what actions you can take to help yourself (and possibly others) reject false information about LGBTQ+ teens, even when they are presented as facts. WW can write your ideas on the lines below.

Please circle the statements below that you think are true and X out the ones you think are false. After you have marked the statements as Myth or Fact, be sure to visit the answer key (in Appendix A under the Activity 14 section) at the back of this workbook and add a * or other symbol of your choosing to indicate which statements are actually factual. Please remember not to judge yourself for any answers you got wrong. As we stated in Activity 7, these activities are not punitive; they are designed to help you grow. It may surprise you to know that even group leaders sometimes have to look up the answers!

Girls who play with trucks when they are young grow up to be lesbians.	LGBTQ+ teens cannot be Christian or join other communities of faith.	Trans kids always tell their parents they are a different gender around age 3.	LGBTQ+ teens are likely just going through a phase they will grow out of later.
LGBTQ+ youth have a heightened risk of suicidal thoughts because they're confused about who they are.	Boys who play with dolls at a young age are probably transgender.	LGBTQ+ teens are highly resilient and able to live happy, fulfilled lives.	Boys grow up gay because their father was absent.
As many as 11.6% of teens identify as LGBTQ+, indicating that it is not rare.	It's harmful to affirm young children who express an LGBTQ+ identity.	LGBTQ+ teens and young adults who get married are more likely to divorce than other couples.	Having just one affirming adult in their life can significantly reduce suicide risk for LGBTQ+ teens.
People who transition from one gender to another are incapable of having biological children.	Most gay and/or trans men contract HIV/AIDS.	LGBTQ+ kids are generally not affected by anti-LGBTQ+ legislation.	Gay boys overidentify with or cling to their mothers and ultimately want to be women.

Step 15: Sources of Information

In Chapter 2 and in the last activity, you were asked to reflect on common myths and facts about LGBTQ+ people. Those activities gave you the chance to identify sources of the information you have gathered about LGBTQ+ teens and/or identify ways to counter inaccurate messages. As you start sorting out which sources are reliable and which sources are not, you may find that you have very few sources of reliable information. That can definitely be the case in rural areas where access to resources, providers, and other parents can be limited (Levine et al., 1975).

When resources are limited, you might consider turning to your LGBTQ+ teen for information. Having an LGBTQ+ teen can make it seem like you have an endless source of insider information. You would not be alone if you ever had the thought, "Who better to ask about gender terminology, trends, and experiences than my teen?" In fact, activities like the erasable dictionary in Chapter 2 require open conversations and consultation with your teenager.

However, we strongly encourage you to proceed with caution. In fact, when we asked community members to comment on early drafts of this workbook, several reviewers (one who ran a group for LGBTQ+ high schoolers) said something like, "Make sure parents do not rely too heavily on their teens for information!"

> You can find additional information about identifying information sources in the Appendix B Activity 15 Scientific Basis paragraph.

They reminded us that LGBTQ+ teens are not experts on all things LGBTQ+. In fact, they are often in the midst of trying to figure themselves out and they may not have a lot of answers. It may go without saying (so please forgive us if this statement seems obvious), but LGBTQ+ teens do not suddenly download a comprehensive encyclopedia on LGBTQ+ identity into their brains the moment they start identifying as LGBTQ+. In many respects, they are just as new to this as you are.

In fact, there are times that you may have more answers than your teen does. As a parent, you are often the best source of information for your child when it comes to a wide range of topics (Riesch et al., 2006). Of course, sexual orientation and gender identity are no exceptions. We certainly encourage you to ask your teen about their personal thoughts, feelings, and experiences. However, we also encourage you to find other sources for general information about LGBTQ+ people (like this workbook). Being a reliable source of information takes planning, and it requires you to establish sources of information you can turn to yourself. The next exercise is designed to help you establish information sources for all sorts of situations.

Activity 15 Information Source List

Below, you will find three information sources. Please fill in the boxes with different types of information that would be appropriate to ask each source. You will notice that the "Ask my Teen" box is smaller than the others. That is to signify that parents are encouraged to look for answers themselves and are discouraged from over relying on their teens as spokespeople for the entire LGBTQ+ community.

Ask Google	Ask a Friend	Ask my Teen

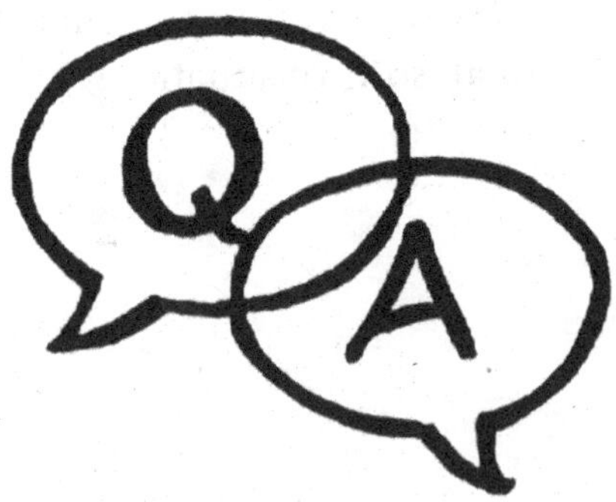

Image 4.2 Information gathering.

Step 16: Looking Ahead to Adulthood

Throughout your teen's life, you have probably thought ahead (with a mix of anticipation and sadness depending on the situation and stage of life) to the future when your teen will grow into an adult. Sometimes you might wish you could "put a brick on their head" to stop them from growing up. At other times, you might dream of a day when your teen will look back on their childhood and finally realize you had their best interest in mind. For better and for worse, your teen will someday be an adult.

The transition from teenage years to adulthood carries with it a whole new range of challenges. In fact, there is growing evidence that the transitional period, the age from 18–25 when a person is on their own for the first time, can take a toll on young adults (Arnett, 2004; Leontopoulou & Delle Fave, 2022). At 18, most teens "age out" of foster care, head off to college, pick up a trade, or otherwise become independent and responsible for their own wellbeing. That process is inherently stressful, but it does not have to be miserable. You can start planning now to support your teen in the present moment in a way that will set them up for success later.

Just like you have packed and unpacked your own baggage during this workshop, it is important for your teen to do the same. We talked in Chapter 1 about how self-exploration and building stronger family relationships can create a strong, protective, healing foundation from which your family can face the world. We want you to experience the benefit that building a healthy family can bring, but we also want to recognize that when you increase your own health, you help people around you (especially your family) become healthier as well (Acton, 2002).

In the opening chapters of this workbook, we talked about self-discovery and effective parenting as a journey. We encouraged you to take care of yourself (stay hydrated) and you prepared to leave behind baggage that could weigh you down. In this exercise, you will be asked to consider what your teen needs for the journey ahead. If you were to pack their backpack for the hike, what would you put in it to help them navigate the transition to adulthood? It might help to look back on your own childhood and ask yourself, "What would I have wanted my own parents to give me to set me up for success?" What are the most valuable things you were given by your caregivers? Bravery? Books? Words of wisdom?

Activity 16 Basic Needs

Take a moment to reflect before you start writing. Make space for any emotions of gratitude, regret, or sadness that surface. Then, in the left column, below, please write down the things you think your child will need to set them up for success for the rest of their lives. On the right column, please write down what you can do to help them acquire what they need. Keep in mind that you have a huge opportunity here to give your teen gifts that will last a lifetime.

Your Teen's Needs	How You Can Meet Those Needs

Bringing It All Together

In this chapter, we took a deep dive into developmental processes and considerations. We asked you to reflect on your own childhood and to think ahead to what your teen might need as they transition to adulthood. Just as we did in previous chapters, we provide an overview of the ways various parents might engage with and work through the content in this chapter. Your experience might be totally different, but if you are working through this book on your own, it can help to gain insight into the experiences and perspectives of other parents relative to your own.

Vignette 7: Mark

In some ways, Mark found Chapter 4 easier to engage with than previous chapters. It felt good to know that he did not do anything to turn his son gay. He could clearly see the ways he tended to think the worst about Devin and then look for evidence in support of his negative perspective. He thought back to when Devin told his mother he was gay and how she immediately assumed Devin would die of AIDS. Just raising his awareness of confirmation bias helped him start to put together a more positive and supportive picture of his son.

However, Mark still faced moments when he felt less engaged with the workbook. He still did not agree with some of the "myth vs. fact" answers and he could recall moments that he had gone to Devin demanding answers about the LGBTQ+ community. As with previous chapters, his progress through the workbook produced a mix of hopeful and frustrating emotions. That was the case when he arrived at the last activity and started reflecting on what he wished his parents had given him to help him get through adulthood. He experienced a lot of sadness when he thought about what he wished his parents had offered him, but was filled with hope about the ways he could support his son in a way he had not been supported himself.

Vignette 8: Kerrie

"Wow," Kerrie thought, as she reviewed the work she'd done in Activity 13, "literally nothing on my graph looks the way I thought it would when I was Dani's age." Kerrie had revisited old aspirations, long-expired crushes, and plans that never quite materialized while completing the activity. She realized that teenage Kerrie was either very optimistic, or completely delusional, and she laughed to herself.

Kerrie realized that Dani, in spite of being a particularly bright student, would probably never go to college. When she reflected on why that had been an important parenting goal for her, she started to see that her parents had left no room for her to not go to college – they practically drilled it into her brain that "after high school comes college," and that's how you succeed in life. When Kerrie read over the Outcomes/Consequences column, she noticed that she generally felt really good about how her life had turned out. Sure, there are things that could be easier (like not having to keep making payments on her student loans), but overall, she felt lucky and happy, even proud of herself.

When Kerrie got home after session 4 of the workshop, Dani was sitting in the living room and the show he was watching had just ended. Dani asked his mom how group went and she said it had gone well and she had taken a humorous trip down memory lane. Dani was eager to hear what Kerrie was referring to when Kerrie offered Dani a deal: "I want to look over this one activity with you first, it asked me to identify what you might need as you transition to adulthood and, honestly, after I wrote down the basics, I wasn't sure what else to put. If you will help me finish this activity, then I will let you read about my adolescent plans for the future, and we can both have a laugh!" Dani couldn't pass up a chance to make fun of his mom for being a dorky teenager and agreed to help her immediately.

Reflection Questions

Image 4.3 A moment to reflect.

- What activity in Module 4 was most challenging for you to complete and why?
- Did you have a lightbulb moment? If so, how would you describe that moment to a friend?
- What are you looking forward to in the next module?
- Over the coming week, notice ways people in your life continue to grow and change as they experience the world.

References

Abreu, R. L., McEachern, A. G., & Kenny, M. C. (2017). Myths and misconceptions about LGBTQ Youth: School counselors' role in advocacy. *Journal of School Counseling, 15*(8). https://eric.ed.gov/?id=EJ1146191

Acton, G. J. (2002). Health-promoting self-care in family caregivers. *Western Journal of Nursing Research, 24*(1), 73–86.

American Academy of Child & Adolescent Psychiatry. (2018). *Conversion therapy.* https://www.aacap.org/aacap/Policy_Statements/2018/Conversion_Therapy.aspx

American Medical Association. (2022). *Advocating for the LGBTQ community.* https://www.ama-assn.org/delivering-care/population-care/advocating-lgbtq-community

American Psychological Association. (2009). *Report of the American Psychological Association task force on appropriate affirmative responses to sexual orientation.* https://www.apa.org/pi/lgbt/resources/therapeutic-response.pdf

Arnett, J. J. (2004). *Emerging adulthood: The winding road from the late teens through the twenties.* Oxford University Press.

Ceatha, N., Koay, A. C. C., Buggy, C., James, O., Tully, L., Bustillo, M., & Crowley, D. (2021). Protective factors for LGBTI+ youth wellbeing: A scoping review underpinned by recognition theory. *International Journal of Environmental Research and Public Health, 18*(21), 11682. https://doi.org/10.3390/ijerph182111682

Cramer, R. J., Golom, F. D., LoPresto, C. T., & Kirkley, S. M. (2008). Weighing the evidence: Empirical assessment and ethical implications of conversion therapy. *Ethics & Behavior, 18*(1), 93–114. https://doi.org/10.1080/10508420701713014

Hafeez, H., Zeshan, M., Tahir, M. A., Jahan, N., Naveed, S., Hafeez, H., Zeshan, M., Tahir, M. A., Jahan, N., & Naveed, S. (2017). Health care disparities among lesbian, gay, bisexual, and transgender youth: A literature review. *Cureus, 9*(4). https://doi.org/10.7759/cureus.1184

Haines, E. L., Deaux, K., & Lofaro, N. (2016). The times they are a-changing . . . or are they not? A comparison of gender stereotypes, 1983–2014. *Psychology of Women Quarterly, 40*(3), 353–363.

Haldeman, D. C. (2022). *The case against conversion "therapy": Evidence, ethics, and alternatives.* American Psychological Association.

Imaz-Sheinbaum, M. (2021). Principles of narrative reason. *History & Theory, 60*(2), 249–270. https://doi.org/10.1111/hith.12205

Kennedy, A. (2024). Intersex. In *Salem Press Encyclopedia*. Salem Press.

Legato, M. (2020). *The plasticity of sex: The molecular biology and clinical features of genomic sex, gender identity and sexual behavior.* Academic Press.

Leontopoulou, S., & Delle Fave, A. (2022). *Emerging adulthood in the COVID-19 pandemic and other crises: Individual and relational resources.* Springer.

Levine, J. M., Samet, M. G., & Brahlek, R. E. (1975). Information seeking with limitations on available information and resources. *Human Factors, 17*(5), 502–513.

Martin, C. L., & Fabes, R. A. (2001). The stability and consequences of young children's same-sex peer interactions. *Developmental Psychology, 37*(3), 431–446. https://doi.org/10.1037/0012-1649.37.3.431

Newcomb, M. E., Feinstein, B. A., Matson, M., Macapagal, K., & Mustanski, B. (2018). "I have no idea what's going on out there:" Parents' perspectives on promoting sexual health in lesbian, gay, bisexual, and transgender adolescents. *Sexuality Research and Social Policy, 15*(2), 111–122. https://doi.org/10.1007/s13178-018-0326-0

Newman, B. M., & Newman, P. R. (2020). *Theories of adolescent development*. Academic Press.

O'Donohue, W. T., Benuto, L. T., & Tolle, L. W. (2013). *Handbook of adolescent health psychology*. Springer.

Pullen Sansfaçon, A., Medico, D., Suerich-Gulick, F., & Temple Newhook, J. (2020). "I knew that I wasn't cis, I knew that, but I didn't know exactly": Gender identity development, expression and affirmation in youth who access gender affirming medical care. *International Journal of Transgender Health, 21*(3), 307–320. https://doi.org/10.1080/26895269.2020.1756551

Riesch, S. K., Anderson, L. S., & Krueger, H. A. (2006). Parent–child communication processes: Preventing children's health-risk behavior. *Journal for Specialists in Pediatric Nursing, 11*(1), 41–56. https://doi.org/10.1111/j.1744-6155.2006.00042.x

Roughgarden, J. (2013). *Evolution's rainbow: Diversity, gender, and sexuality in nature and people* (1st ed.). University of California Press.

Schneider, N. (2021). Stigmatization. In *Encyclopedia of autism spectrum disorders* (pp. 4635–4636). Cham: Springer International Publishing.

Sommer, V., & Vasey, P. L. (2006). Homosexual behaviour in animals: Topics, hypotheses and research trajectories. In V. Sommer, & P. L. Vasey (Eds.), *Homosexual behaviour in animals: An evolutionary perspective* (pp. 3–42). Cambridge University Press.

Tarantino, M. R., & Jamison, T. B. (2023). Resilience through relationship experiences: A qualitative exploration of lesbian, gay, and bisexual romantic development. *LGBTQ+ Family: An Interdisciplinary Journal, 19*(5), 351–366. https://doi.org/10.1080/27703371.2023.2212621

Testa, R. J., Habarth, J., Peta, J., Balsam, K., & Bockting, W. (2015). Development of the gender minority stress and resilience measure. *Psychology of Sexual Orientation and Gender Diversity, 2*(1), 65–77. https://doi.org/10.1037/sgd0000081

Willner, G. (1968). The role of anxiety in obsessive compulsive disorders. *The American Journal of Psychoanalysis, 28*(1), 201–211.

CHAPTER 5

COMING OUT

Making Safe(r) Spaces and Growing Your Affirming Family

Coming Out

Coming out, or telling someone about their LGBTQ+ identity, can be a difficult experience for teens and (by extension) for their families (D'amico et al., 2015; Denes & Afifi, 2014). Teens often fear coming out because they know that the consequences of telling others they are LGBTQ+ can be very hurtful in the short term (Johnson et al., 2020). Some parents disown their LGBTQ+ teens, kick them out of the house, withdraw financial support, or even physically assault their teens (Brown et al., 2020; DeChants et al., 2022). For these reasons, coming out or interacting with other people can be highly stressful for LGBTQ+ teens. As discussed earlier, when a teen's body looks different than their gender identity or when they feel forced to hide who they are, they can feel like they stand out and can have a hard time connecting with others.

However, coming out can also be a positive experience. Disclosing their identities is a first step toward teens living a more connected and less stressful life. Some parents are very encouraging and affirming. Teens who receive family support after coming out may experience increases in self-esteem, gender euphoria, and overall physical and mental health outcomes (Ceatha et al., 2021; McConnell et al., 2016; Medico et al., 2020; Ryan et al., 2009).

Whereas some teens stay "in the closet" or decline to tell others about their identity for fear of being different, other teens out themselves with passion and seem to embrace being part of the LGBTQ+ community. Other teens may come out in stages. For example, a teen may come out as bisexual and then later come out as gay. It is important to allow teens to come out at their own pace and not to jump to conclusions about their identities. For example, it can be hurtful to hear a parent say, "I bet this is just a phase," or "At least he is gay and not transgender." Parents sometimes wonder if their child is identifying as nonbinary, for example, because it is a popular trend or an opportunity to belong to a community. Of course, it is within the realm of possibility that a teen would identify as LGBTQ+ because they think it is cool, but such cases are exceedingly rare for several reasons:

1. Being LGBTQ+ is not easy. If identity were a choice, people would be unlikely to give up their privilege or pick a marginalized group to join. Instead of assuming your teen is being disingenuous, consider acknowledging their bravery and the trust it took to share their identity.
2. It is hard to pretend to be LGBTQ+. Imagine trying to identify as a gender or express an attraction that is not real for you. For example, if you are straight, could you romantically kiss someone with the same gender identity as you? Instead of searching for evidence that your teen is mistaken, consider looking for evidence of their health and well-being.
3. LGBTQ+ people are real and authentic. Suggesting that LGBTQ+ people fabricate identities reinforces age-old myths about LGBTQ+ people being sneaky, frightening, and out to get straight people. Instead, try to look past the beliefs you may have about LGBTQ+ people and see your child for the beautiful, valuable, and genuine person you have always known them to be.

DOI: 10.4324/9781003678205-5

Regardless of why and when teens come out, the truth is that teens are not the only ones who face backlash throughout the coming out process – their families struggle too (Gray et al., 2016; Morgan et al., 2023; Pullen Sansfaçon et al., 2015). Just as LGBTQ+ people get blamed for their identities and questioned about their sanity, so do their parents. In fact, for a long time, LGBTQ+ identity was believed to be the result of (overbearing/overly nurturing/distant) parenting. These kinds of negative ideas and beliefs mean that explaining your teen's LGBTQ+ identity to other people may not be easy. However, having an LGBTQ+ child can also open up opportunities for personal growth and incredible moments of joy. Some parents find rich connections to other parents with LGBTQ+ kids, draw hope from supporting the LGBTQ+ community, and celebrate their own bravery and success as parents (Gray et al., 2016; Matsuno et al., 2022; Morgan et al., 2023).

In this chapter, we will look at boundary-setting and consider ways to prioritize giving your teen the space they need to learn and grow into the authentic human they are and to be proud of their LGBTQ+ identity as one part of their personhood. Because the coming out process can be stressful for your teen and you, we will also look at how the brain processes information during times of stress/crisis and how you can help yourself and others to manage emotions. As you work through this module, remember that your teen holds the final say on when and with whom they share their LGBTQ+ identity.

It is important for safety and autonomy that an LGBTQ+ person is not forced to "out themselves" in a situation where they, for any reason, prefer not to share their identity with others. Even if your teen only wants you to know for now, that's okay and we strongly recommend that you respect their wishes. We think it's important that you spend some time reviewing this module with your teen before you take action or share their identity as a member of the LGBTQ+ community with others.

Step 17: Navigating Family, Schools, and Community

Coming out impacts all levels of a person's life. LGBTQ+ teens face a wide range of resource access barriers (in education, health care settings, and so on) that start before they come out and do not get any better after they do (e.g., Koch & Knutson, 2016). For example, coming out can result in difficult family conversations about who should know about your teen's LGBTQ+ identity, tough realizations about what your community has (or does not have) to support and affirm LGBTQ+ people, and even questions about how school faculty/staff and peers will treat your teen. We hope the next activity will help you think through the process and make decisions, with your teen, that will best meet the needs of your teen and your family.

As you prepare to engage in this activity, please remember:

- Each decision in this activity must be discussed with your teen before you take action.
- This plan can be changed at any time to reflect current realities.
- Take time to learn about any safety measures and resources that may already be in place at school and in your community.
- Some people may be unsure of how to help your teen. Humans tend to have deeply held beliefs, some of which may be helpful and others may be harmful.
- Be concrete and specific about what is needed and acceptable. You can hold people accountable for observable actions, not their thoughts, attitudes, or feelings.
- Some communities will be more difficult to navigate than others.
- You may need to get creative in establishing safe spaces for your teen and other LGBTQ+ people.

Once you've thought about with whom you should or should not share your teen's LGBTQ+ identity, we think it can be helpful to map out your thoughts and concerns. Please remember that this is a collaborative process that can include multiple stakeholders (that is why the pronoun "we" is used throughout the next activity). That does not mean, however, that your needs and experiences have to take a back seat. Your perspectives are valid, important, and are worthy of being recognized (even when you are actively making space for the needs and perspectives of others).

> We further discuss the importance of collaboration in the Appendix B Activity 17 Scientific Basis paragraph.

Activity 17 Collaborative Disclosure Planning

Please use the spaces in the following activity to organize your thoughts and record your teen's input. You can work together to complete the worksheet or ask your teen to review your completed worksheet and place a "√" (check mark) by ideas they agree with and an "X" (cross out) by the ideas they don't agree with.

We are Concerned About Telling . . .	Potential Costs or Unwanted Outcomes . . .	Possible Benefits/Ideal Outcomes . . .

Now that you've thought through with whom you and your teen will share their LGBTQ+ identity; you've identified concerns and considered possible outcomes, we'd like you to explore resources that may already be in place in your community (you may also wish to list resources that are accessible online or in other communities nearby).

Our Community Resource List

Most Trusted Mental Health Provider Near Us:__________________________

Most Trusted Medical Provider Near Us:______________________________

Nearest Active Section of PFLAG is:_________________________________

Most Accepting Faith Community in My Area:__________________________

Most Trusted School Official:______________________________________

My Favorite LGBTQ+ YouTube Channel:_____________________________

My Favorite LGBTQ+ Book/Workbook:_______________________________

The LGBTQ+ Movie I Rely on Most:________________________________

Step 18: Navigating Health Care

Entire books have been written about health care for LGBTQ+ youth (e.g., Magalhães et al., 2022) and ways to provide affirming care for LGBTQ+ people more broadly (e.g., Knutson et al., 2022). It is impossible for us to cover all of the issues, barriers, strategies, and outcomes related to LGBTQ+ health care within this text. Still, there are basic strategies you can use to connect your teen to the care they need.

The first step is to get support for yourself and your teen. Getting medical care can take a very long time and can be incredibly challenging. Given the incredibly high suicide rate among LGBTQ+ youth (Ream, 2022), it is a good idea to get mental health support while you try to sort out the rest of your child's health care needs. Sadly, the availability of national resources for LGBTQ+ people can increase or decrease based on fluctuations in overall attitudes toward LGBTQ+ people, changes in state and federal administrations, and so on. We have included some national resources that were available when this book was published, but you may need to search for more current contacts and/or confirm that the contact information we provided is still accurate. Here are some places to start:

- *In a pressing crisis, calling 911 or proceeding to an emergency room is the primary recommended approach to securing the safety of your teen.* If your teen is at immediate risk for suicide, you can get rapid help by calling 911 or proceeding to the nearest emergency room.
- The Trevor Project offers Chat, Text, and Phone-Based Support: 866-488-7386
- The Trans Lifeline offers Phone-Based Support: 877-565-8860
- The National Suicide and Mental Health Crisis Line (988) also offers text and phone-based support, but it receives government funds and (as of July 17, 2025) is no longer allowed to offer specialized services to LGBTQ+ youth.

If you are preparing for possible future emergencies, you may want to take time to think about which local and national resources are safe to use and create a response plan, especially if you are located in a state that targets parents of trans and nonbinary youth (see Knutson et al., 2025)

> We talk more about a "hope for the best, plan for the worst" approach in the Appendix B Activity 18 Scientific Basis paragraph.

It is also good to know some of the warning signs to look for that may indicate a person is thinking about suicide, such as talking about being a burden to others or feelings of humiliation (Gorse, 2022; Van Orden et al., 2010). A person who feels a lack of connectedness to others and their community or who has experienced physical or sexual abuse or childhood trauma may also have a heightened risk of suicide attempt or completion. We encourage you to review additional warning signs, risk factors, and protective factors in the resource section at the back of this workbook.

The second step is to educate yourself. Unfortunately, many providers are unaware of the current standards of care for LGBTQ+ teens. You and your teen may have to advocate for appropriate care and the first step toward doing so is to understand best practice. For example, if you are the parent of a trans or gender expansive child, you might benefit from reading parts of the World Professional Association for Transgender Health (WPATH) Standards of Care 8th Edition (Coleman et al., 2022). At the very least, you have the right to expect that your teen will be respected and valued.

The third step is to identify any challenges that will come up when you ask for care and what your response will be. For example, if a provider says, "I can't provide gender affirming care for your teenager because it is illegal," how will you respond? We encourage you to stay current regarding legislation in your area as well as on a federal level so you can be confident when you advocate for your teen's medical care and to help you seek providers in areas where the care your teen needs is accessible.

The fourth step is to get creative. While you are navigating the health care system (facing challenges and responding), you may be able to find alternative ways to solve your problems. Within local legal parameters, there may be appropriate resources and organizations that help with transportation or financial resources to obtain affirming healthcare for your teen.

Activity 18 Preparing for Health Care Engagement

Now that you have reflected on the key steps in advocating for your teen, we would encourage you to set a healthcare navigation plan you can reference when working with health service providers such as physicians, psychologists, and others. To do so, you can follow the steps below. Please remember to return to this worksheet as you learn new information or discover new strategies. Like many other worksheets in this workbook, this is intended to be a "living document" that expands and morphs to meet your family's ongoing needs.

Step 1a. List a few behaviors, statements, or other indicators you notice when your teen is experiencing high levels of distress and may need immediate care:

____

____

Step 1b. Identify at least one resource you can access to connect your teen with rapid (or immediate) care (please remember to confirm that the resource is available, accessible, and safe):

____

Step 2. List two or three policy-based truths related to your teens care that you are absolutely confident about (such as "Identity-affirming mental health care is not illegal." or "Based on WPATH Standards of Care, there is nothing disordered or wrong about identifying as nonbinary; nonbinary people are healthy and whole."):

____

____

____

Step 3. List a few challenging responses you expect to get from health service providers and jot down possible responses to the challenges that might raise.

____

____

____

Step 4. Now that you have reflected on risks, sources of support, policies, and challenges, list some creative solutions you can use to meet your teen's health care needs when typical sources of support fall through.

____

____

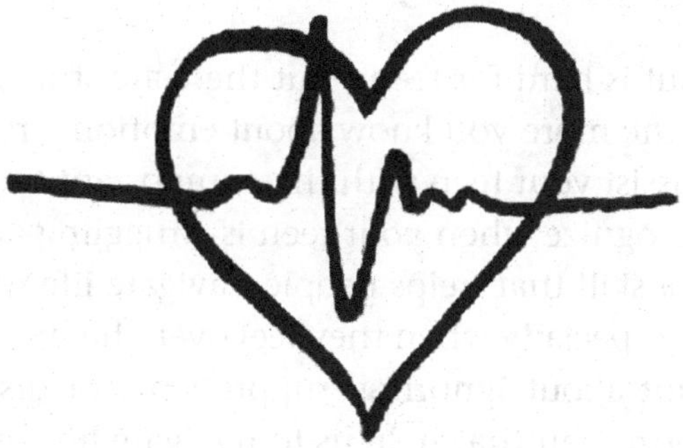

Image 5.1 Toward calming strategies.

Step 19: Brain Basics and Emotion Regulation

We keep saying that coming out is hard for teens, but there are strategies that teens can use to manage hard experiences. As a parent, the more you know about emotional regulation and brain development, the better you can model and assist your teen with these important life skills (see Siegel & Payne Bryson, 2011). You can also learn to recognize when your teen is struggling and better handle stressful interactions. Emotional regulation is a skill that helps people navigate life with other people and it helps you work with your own emotions, especially when they feel overwhelming or intense (Roskam et al., 2023).

Emotional regulation is not about ignoring, suppressing, or dismissing emotions. Emotions are valid, powerful sources of information that help us to navigate life, and sometimes they can get in the way of growth.

> Are you curious about why we added this section to the workbook? You can take a deeper dive by reading the Appendix B Activity 19 Scientific Basis paragraph.

For example, think back to our hiking metaphor – What if you encountered a snake on the trail and experienced intense fear? In this context, most people would agree that fear is an appropriate response. Now imagine that the fear you experienced was so intense that every time you walk outside you are overwhelmed with a fear of snakes. Emotional regulation and support can help you work through this fear and get back out on the trails.

The first step to understanding emotional regulation is to understand the basics of how human brains process information and respond to threats. Below, you will see a basic diagram of the human brain with parts of the brain labeled. As you take a moment to examine the diagram, try to visualize where the parts of the brain are located in your head and imagine feeling them come to life while you read about their functionality. The key parts of the brain that we discuss in this chapter are the:

- Brain Stem: Located at the base of the brain, connects the brain to the spinal cord. The most primitive part of the brain, responsible for autonomic functions such as heartbeat and breathing.
- Amygdala: A small, almond-shaped part of the brain located just above the ear. Used to process emotions, especially fear and anxiety. Fight, flight, freeze response lives in the amygdala.
- Prefrontal Cortex: Located at the front of the head. Responsible for higher thinking skills and organization. Logic and decision making live in the cortex.

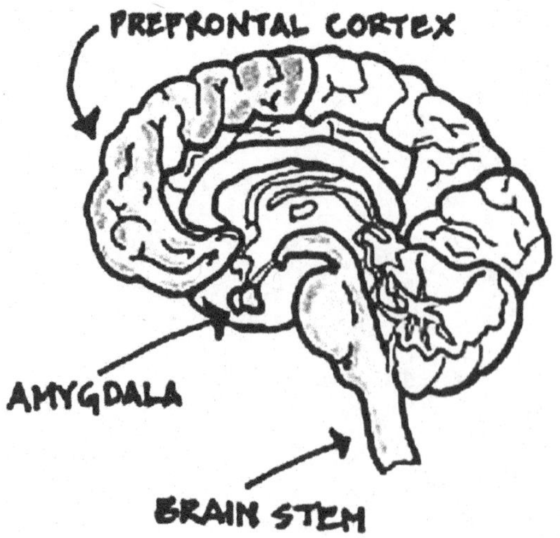

Image 5.2 Brain basics.

Activity 19 Applying Regulation Strategies to Your Family

Now we can apply this model to experiences you may have with your teen. Think of a time your teen seemed emotionally dysregulated and write a brief description below. (For example, you might have asked your teen to go to the grocery store with you and then witnessed them "having a meltdown" because they "can't handle" being in public where people might "make fun of them.")

____

____

____

____

The "meltdown" or moment of dysregulation you witnessed occurred because of processes in your teen's brain. When a person feels threatened (due to real or perceived danger) the amygdala is activated and the prefrontal cortex goes offline. This means that a person who is in a heightened state of arousal (a meltdown) is not able to think logically, has limited ability to consider options and access coping tools; their focus is on survival rather than social norms or expectations. Thinking about the example you wrote down above, what signs were present that your teen might have been operating from the amygdala? Try to think of at least two or three signs such as: they stopped listening, they were sobbing, or their eyes got really wide and they froze.

____

____

Now write down behaviors you would expect your teen to be capable of if their prefrontal cortex were engaged. For example, they might be able to make eye contact, talk things through with you or think of possible solutions to their stressor. Again, please try to think of two or three behaviors or signs.

____

____

Now write down some strategies you could use to help your teen move from operating out of their amygdala to engaging their prefrontal cortex and, in doing do, to become more emotionally regulated. (If you are unsure, visit the calming and coping skills section at the back of this workbook.)

____

____

____

Step 20: Creating Safety to Navigate Emotional Crises

Now that you've learned a little bit about the parts of the brain used for emotional regulation, you can use that knowledge as a foundation to develop even more strategies to help your teen regulate even in very difficult or complex situations. Much of what we have covered in the workbook so far serves as a basic knowledge base you can use to support your teen, build trust, and express meaningful and effective care (not to mention building your own confidence and feelings of effectiveness as a parent). As you near the end of the workbook, you have the opportunity to start integrating what you have learned into more adaptive or creative solutions to meeting your teen where they are. In other words, the work does not stop when you turn the last page of this book. Parenting is a life-long process of discovery and adaptation. We hope you continue to build a toolkit of strategies long after your teen transitions to adulthood.

One area where more advanced or combined/integrative strategies are needed is in the realm of emotional development and emotion regulation. Working with emotions requires the development of an "emotional vocabulary." If you have worked with a therapist before, you might have seen them use a "feelings wheel" or "feelings list" to help you identify and process your emotions. When we talk about emotion regulation, though, we are usually talking about dealing with feelings on the "distressing" or "uncomfortable" end of the emotional spectrum. Emotion regulation is typically needed when a person experiences an emotional crisis or traumatic event.

Emotional crises and traumatic events typically arise when teens feel out of control. By definition, emotional trauma arises when someone feels threatened and out of control of their environment and responds like a cornered animal (such as a turtle or squirrel) by trying to fight, run away (flight), or by freezing (Schultz et al., 2016). As you read this, it is probably easy for you to think of several examples of times your teen acted out of emotional crisis or a trauma response by: becoming angry or aggressive (fight); running to their room and slamming their door (flight); or disengaging and appearing hollow or despondent (freeze). To be clear, we are not saying that every emotional crisis is emotionally traumatic, but there is evidence that LGBTQ+ people develop trauma-like responses to repeated threats, discrimination, and distress (see Urban et al., 2022).

When your teen is emotionally activated (crying, shutting down, or having an angry outburst), it can feel overwhelming and can cause you to become emotionally destabilized or dysregulated yourself.

> We talk a little more about parent responses to dysregulation in the Appendix B Activity 20 Scientific Basis paragraph.

It is hard to stay calm when faced with an emotional hurricane, but it is possible. The trick is not to be drawn into the activation to the point that you become activated too. One strategy is to think of your teen as a turtle and of yourself as their support, healing, example, light, and love (SHELL).

Step 1 toward becoming a SHELL for your teen is conceptualizing your role and reminding yourself of your "job" when times get tough. As a shell, your primary job is to create safety or offer protection, not reaction. That job requires accepting your limits. You cannot protect your teen from every potential harm (and that is not your job as a parent). Even when their SHELL is intact and functioning properly, their appendages can be exposed and there's a softer underside that can be damaged easily. You can, however, protect them from some forms of harm, and you can provide your teen with a safe place to heal when wounded by the outside world. Consider these five steps you can take to help your teen.

Step 2 of becoming a SHELL is engaging in your own healing or emotion regulation. If you have ever flown on an airplane, you know you are supposed to put on your oxygen mask before you assist other passengers with theirs. The best way to get through a crisis is to use your own emotional regulation skills to remain a calm, stable place where your teen can feel safe (Holodynski & Kärtner, 2023). A turtle will not emerge from its shell if someone is yelling or knocking on the shell – it needs a safe environment to emerge and engage.

Step 3 is to model stability for your teen or to set an example through your own responses and behaviors. As your teen's shell, you can offer them the same coping and regulation skills that you are using in a given moment to help them grow emotionally and build resilience for when they encounter hurtful and stressful situations on their own. Your teen learns from watching you, especially when things get hard. You can use that to your advantage.

Step 4 of becoming a SHELL is to illuminate the situation just like a lamp that suddenly comes on in a dark room. In the last section, we pointed out that a person who is emotionally activated is not usually capable of problem solving and may not be able to communicate effectively (their prefrontal cortex is offline; Rutherford, 2023). Therefore, a shell will approach the person calmly, thoughtfully, and without a sense of urgency; instead of focusing on fixing the problem right away. They will first light a path to deescalation that allows for deeper conversation later.

Step 5 is to lay a foundation of love. Becoming emotionally dysregulated is a risky, vulnerable, and often scary experience. After an emotional outburst, teens may experience a "vulnerability hangover" or become afraid that they will be abandoned because they are too difficult, unpleasant to be around, or just "too much" in general. It can be deeply healing for a person to be accepted as who they are, "warts and all." When you express love for your teen after an emotional crisis, it not only shows them that you accept them at a deeper level, it also helps them regulate in the future by rewarding them (in a sense) for stabilizing. That is behaviorism 101: if you get a candy bar (or love) after you do something, you are more likely to do it again.

Activity 20 Cultivating Safe(r) Spaces

Being a SHELL is easier said than done. It takes self-awareness, determination, and practice. A consistent theme in this book is that affirming parenting is grounded in knowing yourself. That principle holds true when it comes to protecting your teen. It is easier to be a SHELL when doing so is a core part of who you are and how you conceptualize your role as a parent. If you think about it, every turtle shell is a little different. The shell fits the needs, size, shape, and environment of the turtle. This activity is designed to help you identify your own unique approach to creating an environment of safety for your teen. Please fill in each of the 5 sections on the turtle's back with your unique shell strategies:

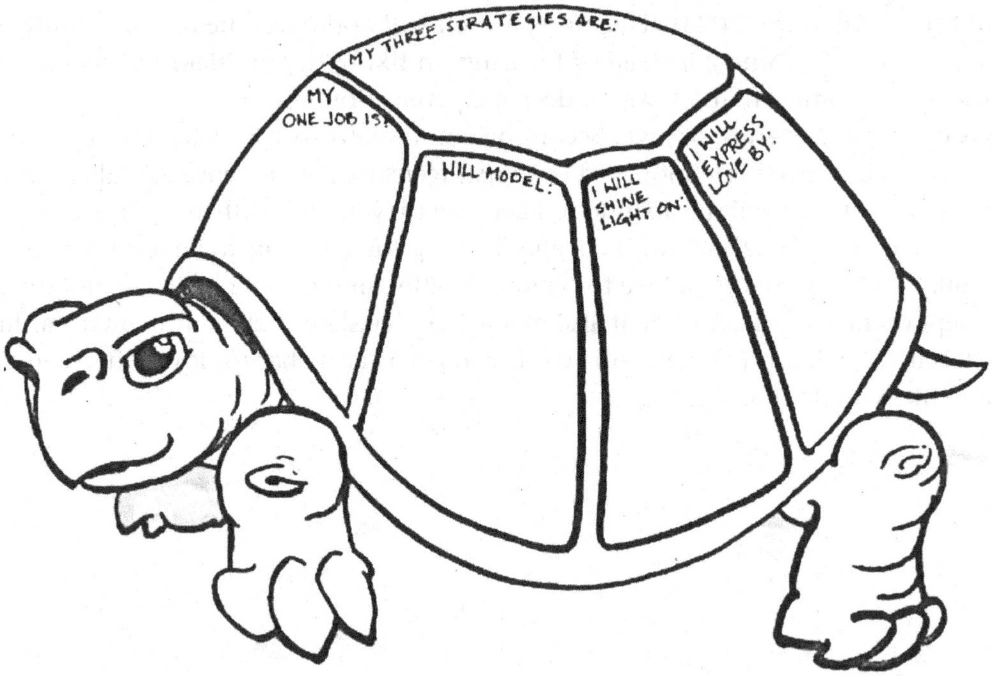

Image 5.3 Shell strategy ideas.

Bringing It All Together

In this chapter, we examined key elements of the "coming out" or identity disclosure process, barriers to medical care, and discussed ways parents can help their teens regulate their emotions. Those processes are inextricably linked because coming out, navigating social spaces, and accessing medical care can be very stressful processes for teens and their families, especially in rural areas. Having emotion regulation strategies is a key to setting LGBTQ+ teens and their families up for success, especially in stressful situations and in the face of emotional crises.

Vignette 9: Mark

Mark always saw himself as his family's protector. Over time, he had learned that his "protector mode" had upsides and downsides. On the upside, it made him the "go-to" guy in the family. When something needed fixing, Mark was the first person they called. On the downside, Mark's "fix it" mindset could get him into trouble, especially when the problem could not be fixed. When his wife started struggling at work and just needed someone to share her struggles with, she would often become frustrated and say, "I don't need someone to fix it! I just need someone to listen!"

For that reason, Mark found the first two activities in Chapter 5 easy to work though. He might not completely agree with Devin's "lifestyle," but the chapter gave him problems he could solve and he liked that. Then the chapter shifted to a discussion of emotions and he started to struggle. Mark started feeling like a "cornered animal" himself as he thought about how helpless people can feel in the midst of an emotional crisis. His need for control and a quick fix started to show up big time.

Then, he started reading about the SHELL principle of emotion regulation and he started to find his feet again. He found it reassuring to know that "every shell is different" and he felt even more grounded when he was able to define his own "job" as a parent for Devin. He confidently wrote "fixer" in the turtle shell activity and started to reflect on ways he could use that identity to ground himself and show up for Devin. He decided he could breathe, have faith, and live by example for his son. For the first time in a long time, he felt like he had something to offer not just Devin, but himself and other people in his life. He committed to being a (more intentional, authentic, and grounded) source of support, healing, light, and love to his son in a way only he could.

Vignette 10: Kerrie

Kerrie was excited to learn more about helping Dani regulate his emotions. She had googled "what to do when your teenager still throws fits" some months ago and read advice about staying calm, refusing to engage until he calms down, and talking about what happened after Dani was in a more regulated state. She tried not to get pulled into Dani's emotions and, nearly every time, she failed. She couldn't stand to see Dani upset and she just wanted to "make it better," and see Dani smile again.

When Kerrie got to class, she wondered if her Google search results would be repeated and, if so, she planned to ask lots of questions about how to make these strategies work. It was helpful when the group talked about the parts of the brain and how they work to manage emotions and stressful situations. She imagined feeling the parts of her brain light-up while the group leader explained their functions and she was surprised to experience a kind of tingly feeling move around her head as the discussion moved from the brain stem to the amygdala and finally to the prefrontal cortex.

Kerrie remembered seeing Dani look back at her with a blank expression one time when a tense conversation between them had turned into a screaming match, and she felt ashamed that she hadn't realized Dani probably *wanted* to respond to her and fix the situation, but he literally couldn't. When Kerrie shared this situation with the group, she was relieved to hear that other parents had made similar mistakes and when the group leader told them, "You can't know what you didn't know until you knew it, so let yourselves off the hook and focus on what you can do differently next time," Kerrie felt assured that, while she couldn't change the past, she could make positive changes for the future.

When she read about being a SHELL for Dani, a light bulb clicked on in Kerrie's brain. She wasn't being a good SHELL; she was suffocating her teen and might even be denying Dani the chance to practice important coping skills that he will need as he navigates life. Kerrie decided that she would work harder to let Dani try to solve his problems, to be more of a sounding board where Dani can bounce ideas off her rather than directing him the way she thinks he should go. Kerrie felt a little nervous about this idea, and she reminded herself that Dani is quickly approaching adulthood, and she decided to focus on her hope that he will be confident in his own ability to solve problems and navigate the world on his own soon.

Reflection Questions

Image 5.4 A moment to reflect.M.

- What activity in Chapter 5 was the most challenging for you to complete? Why?
- Did you have a lightbulb moment? How would you describe that moment to a friend?
- What are you looking forward to in the next chapter?
- Over the next week, identify and practice at least one calming skill. Consider inviting your teen to join you.

References

Brown, C., Porta, C. M., Eisenberg, M. E., McMorris, B. J., & Sieving, R. E. (2020). Family relationships and the health and well-being of transgender and gender-diverse youth: A critical review. *LGBT Health, 7*(8), 407–419. https://doi.org/10.1089/lgbt.2019.0200

Ceatha, N., Koay, A. C. C., Buggy, C., James, O., Tully, L., Bustillo, M., & Crowley, D. (2021). Protective factors for LGBTI+ youth wellbeing: A scoping review underpinned by recognition theory. *International Journal of Environmental Research and Public Health, 18*(21), 11682. https://doi.org/10.3390/ijerph182111682

Coleman, E., Radix, A. E., Bouman, W. P., Brown, G. R., de Vries, A. L. C., Deutsch, M. B., . . . Arcelus, J. (2022). Standards of care for the health of transgender and gender diverse people, version 8. *International Journal of Transgender Health, 23*(sup1), S1–S259. https://doi.org/10.1080/26895269.2022.2100644

D'amico, E., Julien, D., Tremblay, N., & Chartrand, E. (2015). Gay, lesbian, and bisexual youths coming out to their parents: Parental reactions and youths' outcomes. *Journal of GLBT Family Studies, 11*(5), 411–437. https://doi.org/10.1080/1550428X.2014.981627

DeChants, J. P., Shelton, J., Anyon, Y., & Bender, K. (2022). "It kinda breaks my heart": LGBTQ young adults' responses to family rejection. *Family Relations, 71*(3), 968–986. https://doi.org/10.1111/fare.12638

Denes, A., & Afifi, T. D. (2014). Coming out again: Exploring GLBQ individuals' communication with their parents after the first coming out. *Journal of GLBT Family Studies, 10*(3), 298–325. https://doi.org/10.1080/1550428X.2013.838150

Gorse, M. (2022). Risk and protective factors to LGBTQ+ youth suicide: A review of the literature. *Child and Adolescent Social Work Journal, 39*(1), 17–28. https://doi.org/10.1007/s10560-020-00710-3

Gray, S. A. O., Sweeney, K. K., Randazzo, R., & Levitt, H. M. (2016). "Am I doing the right thing?": Pathways to parenting a gender variant child. *Family Process, 55*(1), 123–138. https://doi.org/10.1111/famp.12128

Holodynski, M., & Kärtner, J. (2023). Parental coregulation of child emotions. In I. Roskam, J. J. Gross, & M. Mikolajczak (Eds.), *Emotion regulation and parenting* (pp. 129–148). Cambridge University Press.

Johnson, K. C., LeBlanc, A. J., Sterzing, P. R., Deardorff, J., Antin, T., & Bockting, W. O. (2020). Trans adolescents' perceptions and experiences of their parents' supportive and rejecting behaviors. *Journal of Counseling Psychology, 67*(2), 156–170. https://doi.org/10.1037/cou0000419

Knutson, D., Goldbach, C., & Koch, J. (2022). *Counseling in a gender expansive world: Resources to support therapeutic practice*. Rowman & Littlefield.

Knutson, D., Soper, J., & Avance, R. (2025). Digital literacy for resistance: Implications for affirming practice with rural TNB youth and their families. *Journal of Health Service Psychology, 51*(2), 64–71.

Koch, J., & Knutson, D. (2016). Transgender clients in rural areas and small towns. *Journal of Rural Mental Health, 40*(3–4), 154–163. https://doi.org/10.1037/rmh0000056

Magalhães, C. L., Sprott, R. A., & Nic Rider, G. (Eds.). (2022). *Mental health practice with LGBTQ+ children, adolescents, and emerging adults in multiple systems of care*. Rowman & Littlefield.

Matsuno, E., McConnell, E., Dolan, C. V., & Israel, T. (2022). "I am fortunate to have a transgender child": An investigation into the barriers and facilitators to support among parents of trans and nonbinary youth. *LGBTQ+ Family: An Interdisciplinary Journal, 18*(1), 1–19. https://doi.org/10.1080/1550428X.2021.1991541

McConnell, E. A., Birkett, M., & Mustanski, B. (2016). Families matter: Social support and mental health trajectories among lesbian, gay, bisexual, and transgender youth. *Journal of Adolescent Health, 59*(6), 674–680. https://doi.org/10.1016/j.jadohealth.2016.07.026

Medico, D., Pullen Sansfaçon, A., Zufferey, A., Galantino, G., Bosom, M., & Suerich-Gulick, F. (2020). Pathways to gender affirmation in trans youth: A qualitative and participative study with youth and their parents. *Clinical Child Psychology and Psychiatry, 25*(4), 1002–1014. https://doi.org/10.1177/1359104520938427

Morgan, H., Wells, L., Lin, A., Strauss, P., & Perry, Y. (2023). Parental challenges, facilitators and needs associated with supporting and accepting their trans child's gender. *LGBTQ+ Family: An Interdisciplinary Journal, 19*(1), 70–86. https://doi.org/10.1080/27703371.2022.2142717

Pullen Sansfaçon, A., Robichaud, M. J., & Dumais-Michaud, A.-A. (2015). The experience of parents who support their children's gender variance. *Journal of LGBT Youth, 12*(1), 39–63. https://doi.org/10.1080/19361653.2014.935555

Ream, G. L. (2022). Trends in deaths by suicide 2014–2019 among lesbian, gay, bisexual, transgender, queer, questioning, and other gender/sexual minority (LGBTQ+) youth. *Journal of Adolescent Health, 71*(5), 609–615. https://doi.org/10.1016/j.jadohealth.2022.06.017

Roskam, I., Gross, J. J., & Mikolajczak, M. (Eds.). (2023). *Emotion regulation and parenting*. Cambridge University Press.

Rutherford, H. J. V. (2023). Neurobiology of parenting and implications for emotion regulation. In I. Roskam, J. J. Gross, & M. Mikolajczak (Eds.), *Emotion regulation and parenting* (pp. 229–243). Cambridge University Press.

Ryan, C., Huebner, D., Diaz, R. M., & Sanchez, J. (2009). Family rejection as a predictor of negative health outcomes in white and latino lesbian, gay, and bisexual young adults. *Pediatrics, 123*(1), 346–352. https://doi.org/10.1542/peds.2007-3524

Schultz, K., Cattaneo, L. B., Sabina, C., Brunner, L., Jackson, S., & Serrata, J. V. (2016). Key roles of community connectedness in healing from trauma. *Psychology of Violence, 6*(1), 42–48. https://doi.org/10.1037/vio0000025

Siegel, D. J., & Payne Bryson, T. (2011). *The whole-brain child: 12 revolutionary strategies to nurture your child's developing mind*. Bantam Books.

Urban, B., Knutson, D., Klooster, D., & Soper, J. (2022). Social-contextual influences on eating pathology in transgender and nonbinary adults. *Eating Disorders: The Journal of Treatment and Prevention*. https://doi.org/10.1080/10640266.2022.2135715

Van Orden, K. A., Witte, T. K., Cukrowicz, K. C., Braithwaite, S. R., Selby, E. A., & Joiner Jr., T. E. (2010). The interpersonal theory of suicide. *Psychological Review, 117*(2), 575–600. https://doi.org/10.1037/a0018697

CHAPTER 6

ADVOCACY

Showing Up for Your LGBTQ+ Child

Advocacy

Congratulations! If you have been completing the chapters in order, you have reached the last section of this workbook. To bring back our hiking metaphor, you may be nearing the summit of the mountain you have been climbing over the course of your engagement with this workbook. We hope you take this chance to look back and see the incredible distance you have traveled.

This is a good time to pause and reflect on your journey so far. You might try to remember the baggage you sorted through, the ways you planned to keep yourself safe, and the depths at which you explored your own identity. You might call to mind the deep love you have for your child. Your thoughts might land on the moments at which you determined to be brave enough to keep going and the times you felt proud to be your child's parent.

It is important to take note of these moments and to acknowledge your accomplishments. Self-care and self-affirmation are crucial parts of this work. If you do not take time to appreciate your accomplishments, few other people will. Caring for ourselves is a key part of mental and emotional resilience and an important skill to model for our teens.

Another part of mental and emotional health is the ability to act in line with your altruistic beliefs and values (Whittingham & Coyne, 2019). In other words, we feel best when we show up for and support the people we love and believe in. That is why this workbook ends with a module on advocacy. As you reach the end of this journey, you may start wondering, "What's next?" or "How can I help my teen now that I feel closer to them and more aligned with their bright future?"

If you are having thoughts about "what's next," you are in the process of realizing that the journey you started in this workshop (or even well before this workshop) is far from over. You have reached an important milestone on this path of love, affirmation, acceptance, and investment, and you know that loving, supporting and parenting a child is a lifelong journey. In other words, you have not reached the top of the mountain, you are just on a plateau. Plateaus give you the chance to look back and marvel at your progress, catch your breath, and rest a bit. A destination has not been reached, rather you're gearing up for the next stretch of the journey.

In truth, there is still a long, hard, rewarding, incredible road ahead of you, and we hope you feel more prepared to celebrate the beauty and the unique opportunities parents of LGBTQ+ children get to experience. Before you embark on that next stage of your parenting journey, we have one last resource to add to your backpack that we believe will set you up for success. That tool is "advocacy" or the capacity to stand up for your LGBTQ+ teen and secure the resources and support they need to be successful.

We will start by helping you explore advocacy as a concept and then we will help you strategize ways to engage in advocacy even when it is hard. To be sure, advocacy can feel scary, especially for people who do not like to stand out or in situations that are likely to result in conflict. That is a common

DOI: 10.4324/9781003678205-6

fear, and we believe it is possible to find advocacy exciting and empowering while taking steps to preserve and observe considerations of safety. This chapter is designed to help you become the advocate you need to be for your child. The good news is that there is no single right way to advocate: You just need to be you and show up for your child.

We truly hope that you eventually find advocacy to be energizing (even if it feels daunting or too contentious at first). The topics we discuss in the next worksheets can be sad, heavy, and difficult to think about. The oppression that LGBTQ+ youth face can be disheartening and painful. We encourage you to remember that your teen is resilient; you are resilient; together, you are equal to the tasks that life may throw your way.

Step 21: Models for Advocacy

There are several models for advocacy designed for nurses, psychologists, sociologists, and other professionals (Earnest et al., 2023; McLaren et al., 2023; Milkman et al., 2010; World Health Organization, 2023). Many of those models use an ecological approach (Bronfenbrenner, 2000) or are based on an understanding that "no person is an island" (e.g., Knutson et al., 2021). In other words, people exist in ecosystems.

This means that each person is nestled (sort of like a nesting doll) in relationships, cultures, social expectations, and so on. Ecological models usually include at least three levels: The Individual Level, The Interpersonal Level, and The Structural Level (Bronfenbrenner, 2000). Effective LGBTQ+ advocacy helps LGBTQ+ teens on each of these levels of their experiences.

Advocacy starts out as an act.

> We talk more about how parents' actions model appropriate behaviors for teens in the Appendix B Activity 21 Scientific Basis paragraph.

You may stand up for your child when someone at the grocery store misgenders them or you may seek out solutions for your child to receive gender affirming care. There are lots of ways you can "do" advocacy. Legislative efforts, serving on your local school board, or assisting your church with increasing affirming practices are some ways to support your teen in your community.

Over time, advocacy becomes a way of life (Whittlesey, 2022; Yep, 2021). The ways you care for and affirm your child can become reflexive, automatic behaviors you don't even think about. We hope that, as you continue the work you started here, you will become the sort of advocate for your teen who never gives up on the idea that the world can grow and embrace LGBTQ+ identities someday. Sometimes we may find allies in unexpected places; advocacy may be simply asking for support or resources that already exist around you. This worksheet will help you plan to have a global impact on the experiences of LGBTQ+ teens. Whenever possible and appropriate, be sure to include your teen in this conversation.

Activity 21 The Advocacy Ecosystem

The Individual Level

The first level of advocacy targets the direct impact a policy or problem has on your LGBTQ+ teen. On the lines below, please write a few things you could do to advocate by working to reduce the impact of discrimination or rejection on your LGBTQ+ teen. For example, you might attend a medical appointment with your teen and make sure the receptionist has the correct pronouns documented in your teen's chart so they are used throughout your teen's medical visit.

____

____

____

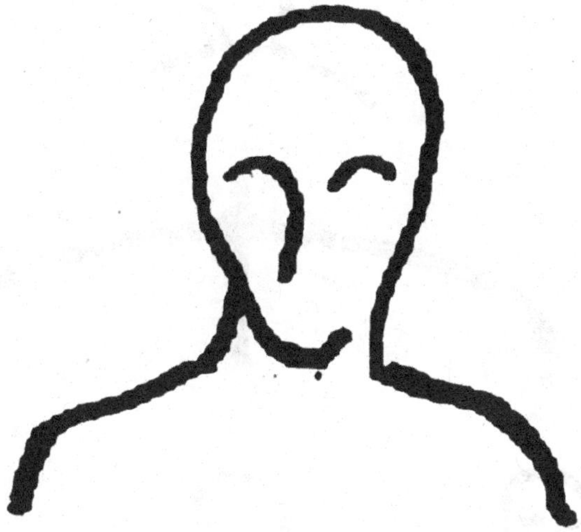

Image 6.1 The individual.

The Interpersonal Level

The second level of advocacy targets the impact of relationships and social connections on your teen. On the lines below, please write down a few things you could do to reduce the negative impact (or increase the positive impact) that others have on your teen. For example, you might ask your teen's teacher to give your teen permission to text you during lunchtime when they are more likely to be bullied and may need to coregulate or connect with you to counteract mounting distress and fear (see Murray et al., 2023).

____

____

____

The Structural Level

The third level of advocacy targets the impact of broader systems, organizations, laws, policies, or rules that impact your teen. On the lines below, please write down a few things you could do to reduce the impact of anti-LGBTQ+ societal dynamics on your teen. For example, you might advocate for a single-user bathroom at your teen's school to reduce exposure to bullying in binary bathrooms and locker rooms.

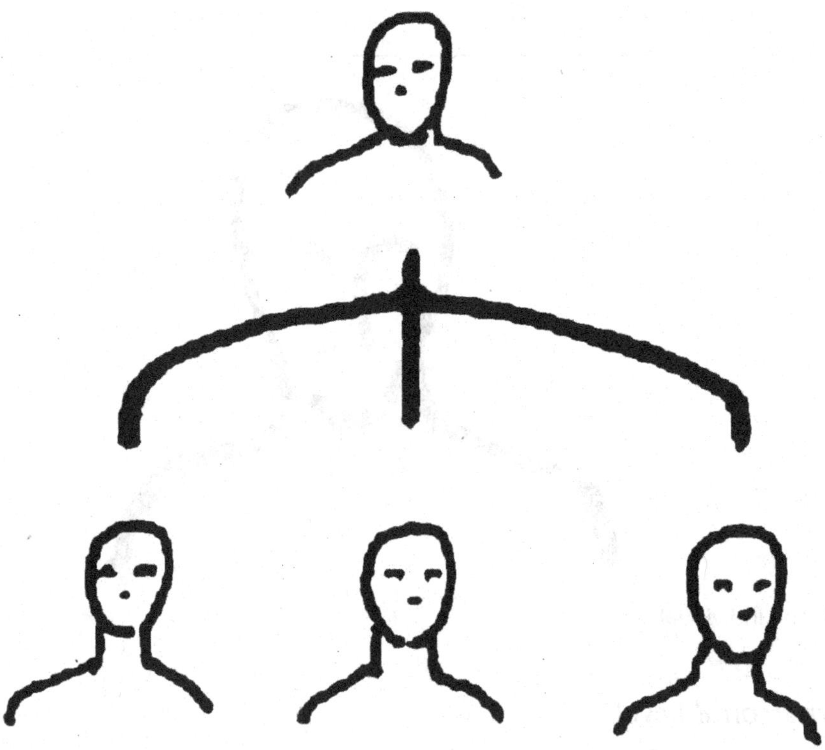

Image 6.2 The ecosystem.

Step 22: Where to Start

As you list out and explore ways to advocate for your teen, you may notice a lot of emotions coming up such as frustration, apprehension, worry, or even a sense of being overwhelmed by all of the changes that need to be made. As we mentioned in the previous section, these feelings regularly come up for advocates and they can hold people back from advocating. What's more, a degree of worry about backlash is valid and reasonable. Fears may get in the way, but they can also keep us safe.

For example, some parents in rural areas have been attacked after supporting their child or trying to help their teen access appropriate health services (see Knutson et al., 2025). We do not want to overstate the risks, but we also want to acknowledge that advocating for your teen can be hard and even scary. There can be pressure to be the "perfect advocate parent" who has absolutely no problem, no regrets, and a deep sense of duty to advocate for all LGBTQ+ youth. Parents can feel guilty or judged if they do not advocate "correctly" every chance they get. If you carry those worries around, we invite you to let them go. In this workbook, we believe parents are more likely to thrive when they stop living in fear of being criticized and start looking for chances to be the best version of themselves. In other words, when it comes to advocacy, there is no judgment, there are just opportunities to show up.

Taking the pressure out of advocacy helps, but it only goes so far. Advocating can still be daunting, anxiety provoking, and conflictual. It is important to observe and respond to fear and anxiety, but when they stop protecting you and start holding you back, they are important to address. One way researchers and therapists have helped LGBTQ+ people get around fear is by using an exposure hierarchy or (in less technical terms) a fear ladder (see Ellard et al., 2010; Knutson et al., 2020). Fear ladders (or exposure hierarchies) break down activities that a person is avoiding and makes them easier to deal with. When things feel difficult, new, or too big to tackle, you can use the "ladder approach" to keep yourself from avoiding important work (Springer & Tolin, 2020).

> We dig deeper into the importance of advocacy in the Appendix B Activity 22 Scientific Basis paragraph.

For example, if your goal is to tell your parents that your teen is LGBTQ+ (and you have your teen's permission to share that information with your parents), but you are fearful about how your parents will respond, you can break the advocacy task down into steps. Your primary task or goal (I will tell my parents that my teen is LGBTQ+ and I am okay with that.) goes at the top of the ladder. Then you can build your steps from the bottom of the ladder until you reach your goal:

- Primary Task/Goal: I will tell my parent that my teen is LGBTQ+ and that I affirm them for who they are.

- Step 3: I will invite my parents to a neutral meeting place like the park in town.

- Step 2: I will plan what I am going to say or even write down a script for the conversation.

- Step 1: I will explore my thoughts and feelings about talking to my parents and identify strategies to regulate my emotions.

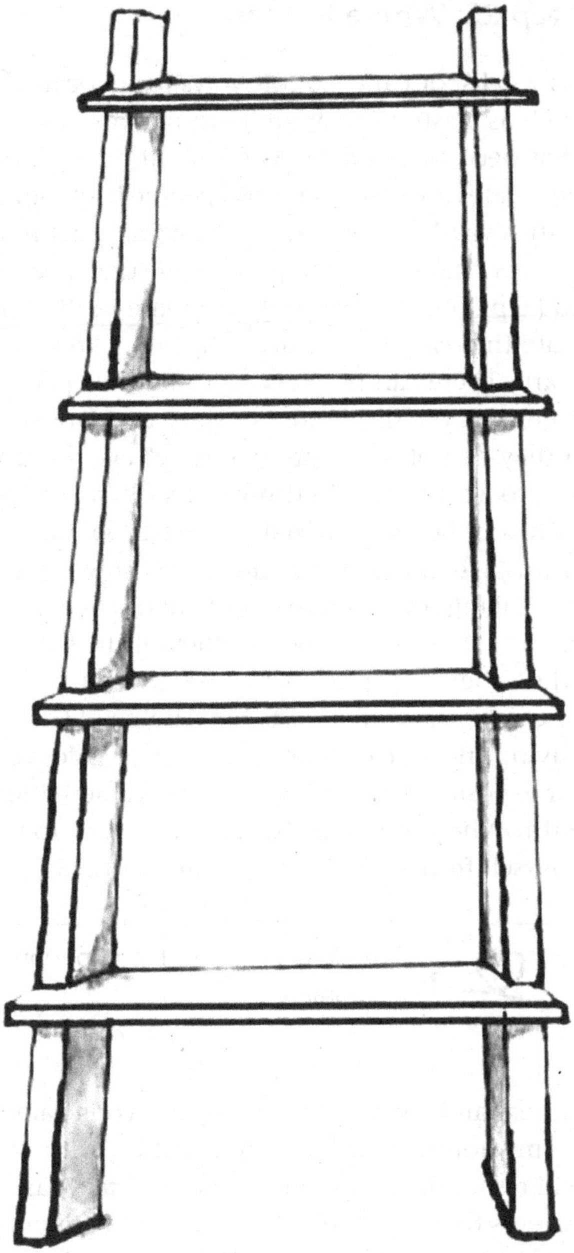

Image 6.3 Ladder example.

Note that the steps build up from the bottom toward the goal that we introduced in the last paragraph. The next activity will lead you through the process of building your own fear ladder.

Activity 22 Steps Toward Advocacy

To use the ladder, start by thinking about one of the advocacy tasks you wrote down on the last worksheet. Then, write a task or goal at the top of the ladder. Next, try breaking that task down into smaller steps, starting at the bottom of the ladder and working your way toward your goal at the top.

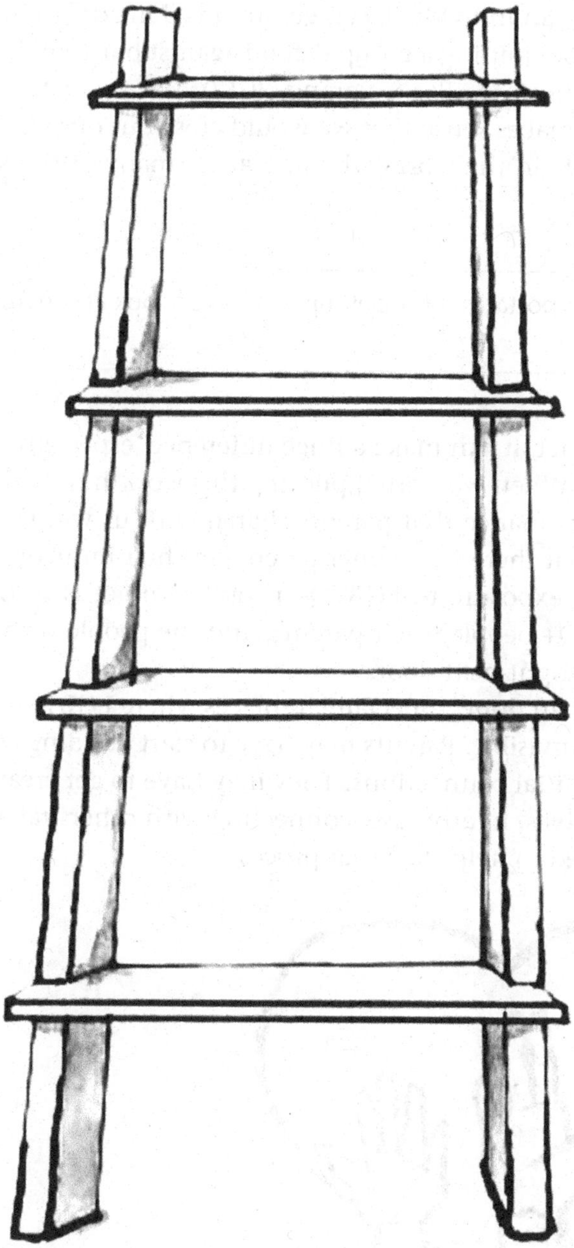

- Primary Task/Goal:
- Step 3:
- Step 2:
- Step 1:

Image 6.4 Your ladder.

Step 23: Getting Involved

Earlier in this workbook, we noted that most health researchers and the affirming care models they recommend include a social support component. In other words, most affirming care models encourage clinicians and advocates to connect LGBTQ+ teens with other LGBTQ+ teens in safe, supportive, and health-fostering environments. That is because, among other reasons, social support is strongly associated with positive health outcomes in LGBTQ+ populations and low levels of social support are associated with poorer health outcomes (McDonald, 2018). That is one of the many reasons we formatted this workbook so that parents could complete it in group settings. Social support matters.

So far, we have focused on ways that you, as an individual, can get involved in advocacy, but there are benefits to group efforts as well. Not only does joining a group defend against burnout, it also helps advocates pool resources and maximize their efforts (Miller & Sprang, 2017). We opened this book by reminding you that you are not alone. It only makes sense that we would close out our work together with the same reminder. There are other people in the world who are facing many of the same challenges and discoveries as you are.

If you need a reminder about the importance of social support, take a look at the Appendix B Activity 23 Scientific Basis paragraph.

While it may seem like a simple statement of fact, it can make a huge difference, especially for parents in rural areas who can feel isolated and alone. When we started piloting this workshop with groups of parents, one of the main benefits of group attendance that parents shared with us was the discovery that they were not alone. It helped to know that there were other parents in their immediate community who had LGBTQ+ teens. When the only exposure to LGBTQ+ people you get is through TV or media, it can be hard to remember that LGBTQ+ people, their parents, and the people who love them are everywhere. In all actuality, they might be right next door.

Still, building a community is easier said than done, especially in places where LGBTQ+ communities and parents of LGBTQ+ people are largely invisible. Parents may have to start building connections online or travel to an urban area to establish initial connections. They may have to get creative, search social media sites, or even start groups themselves. In any case, connecting with others takes planning and intentionality. The next activity is designed to help start that process.

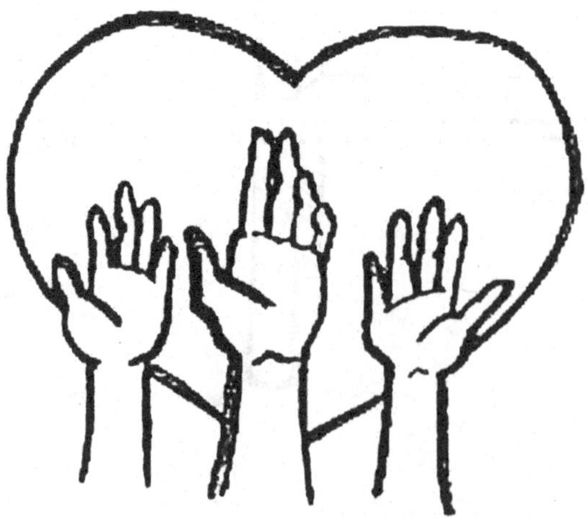

Image 6.5 Becoming an advocate.

Activity 23 Building an Advocacy Network

Below is a list of options for advocacy and community involvement. Please place an "X" next to any groups you plan to contact. Then conduct your own search for options and write any groups you find on the blank lines. If you plan to start a group yourself, you can write that plan on one of the blank lines as well.

___ The Local Youth Services Advisory Board

___ The Nearest PFLAG Chapter

___ The Local High School GSA (Gender and Sexuality Alliance)

___ The Parent-Teacher-Association (PTA)

___ An Open and Affirming Church

___ A Parenting Group at the Local Library

___ A Social Media Group for LGBTQ+ People in your Area

____

____

____

____

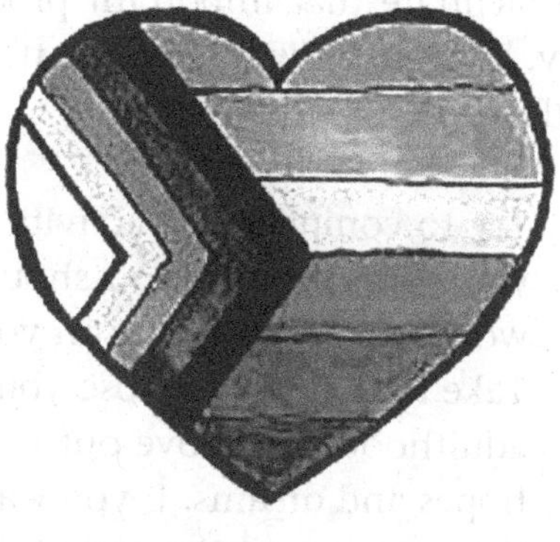

Image 6.6 Love and pride.

Step 24: Revisiting Your Dream

This activity is a bit of a departure from the other activities in the book. So far, in each section of this book we have introduced new concepts, approaches, and exercises that build on each other and expand the tools you have at your disposal. We hope you will continue that work on your own. There is a lot left for you to discover, and there is no way we could cover everything in one book.

However, before we say "goodbye," we hope to bring you full circle.

> Goodbyes can be hard so we provided additional information and reflection opportunities in the Appendix B Activity 24 Scientific Basis paragraph.

In the opening chapter of this book, we asked you to set goals for yourself and we noted that goal-setting sets people up for success in therapeutic settings (Epton et al., 2017) and beyond. However, goals do more than just serve as a north star to guide your progress through the journey of discovery. They also help you realize how much progress you have made when you reach the end of the journey (or at least the benchmark of a plateau that gives you a chance to look back down the mountain and recalibrate your focus on the peak).

To facilitate that important process of reflection and re-centering, we will not introduce a new activity. Instead, we will return to the very beginning. Before you complete the next activity, please do the following:

- Try to complete the activity without revisiting or thinking about your answers the first time you completed it. You should approach it as the parent you are now, after completing the workbook, not the person you were when you started.
- Take a moment to close your eyes and reflect on what you want for your teen as they enter adulthood and move out into the world on their own. Focus on the most important pieces, hopes and dreams. If you want to reflect more before completing the activity, you can skip to the questions at the end of this chapter and then come back to the activity.
- Do your best to suspend any judgments or critical voices in your head. This dream is yours and that is okay. You do not have to dream someone else's dream.

Now move to the activity and write your reflections in the space provided.

Activity 24 A Dream Revisited

Please record the dream(s) you have for your LGBTQ+ teen, especially as it relates to relationships and life achievements.

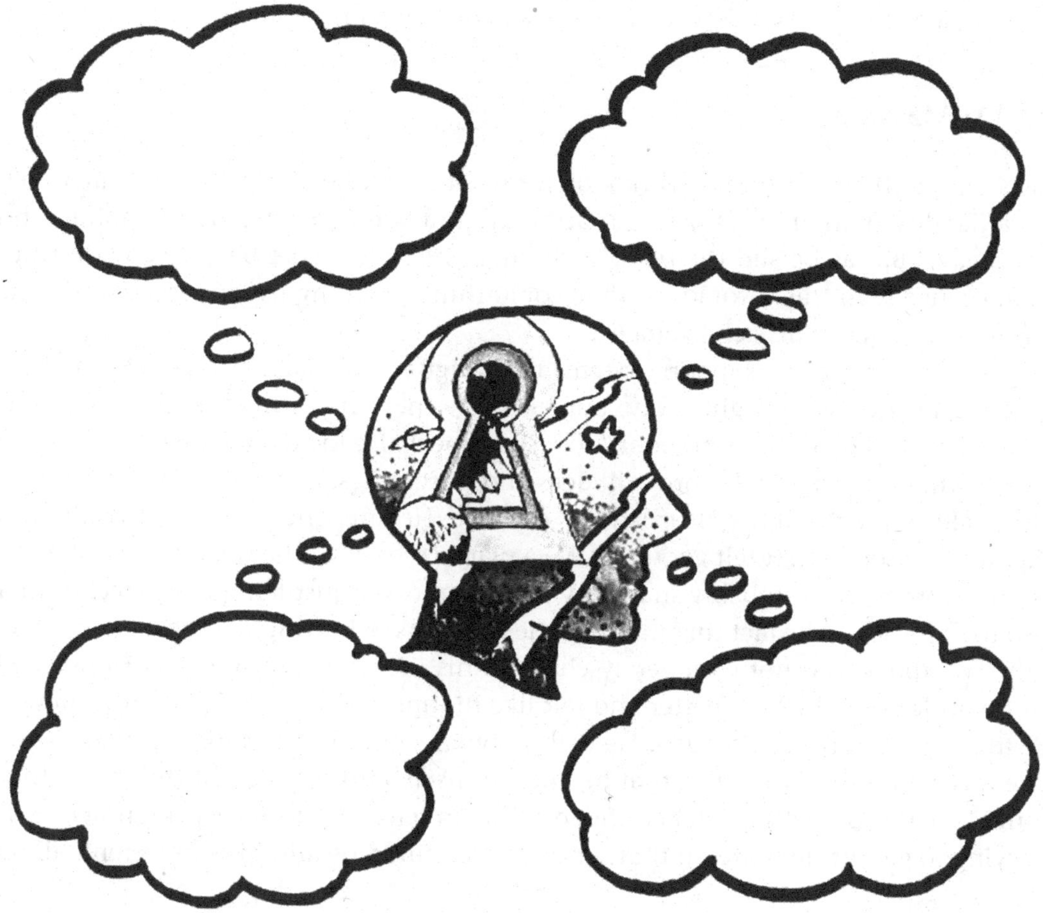

Image 6.7 Parenting dreams revisited.

Take a moment to look back over your dream and compare it to the dream activity you completed at the beginning of this workshop.

- What has changed?
- What has not changed?
- What do you make of the differences and similarities?

Bringing It All Together

In this chapter, we dug into the process and specifics of advocacy. We started by exploring the different levels of advocacy (individual, interpersonal, and systemic), and we identified barriers to advocacy such as fear and anxiety. Then we offered strategies to work through barriers and examined the benefits of community connection. Finally, we returned to the very first activity in the workbook and reflected on ways our dreams for our LGBTQ+ teens changed and stayed the same.

Vignette 11: Mark

Mark slowly closed the cover on his workbook for what might be the last time. Sometimes he viewed it more as a liability than an asset, given that he did not want to get caught reading a resource that seemed "pro-gay." But as he slid the book back under his side of the bed, he couldn't help feeling a little proud. He had seen this through, and he could think of a long list of people who wouldn't have. It was impossible to ignore his achievement.

It felt good to think about support systems that might be available to him. He didn't see himself jumping into a PFLAG group right away, but he knew there had to be other people out there who "would make it to the end of the workbook" too, so to speak. He looked forward to finding more people like him with whom he could talk through ideas and misgivings.

He also really appreciated the "fear ladder" exercise. He knew he would eventually need to talk to his wife about their son, and it felt good to have a plan. To be clear, he wasn't afraid, but it was nice to know that his worries were probably shared by other parents. It just felt good to feel normal.

He also took solace in the fact that many of the elements of his original dream had stayed the same. Reading the workbook had not completely changed his life or his perspective. He was still the same Mark, but he understood himself better and felt like his approach to his family was more intentional. That isn't to say that nothing changed. He definitely knew more about his son than when he started out, but he was comforted by the fact that he knew himself a little better. At the end of the day, he felt like he could love his son with greater confidence. Devin felt less like a scary unknown and more like a teen just trying to get through life. In that sense, Mark figured he and his son weren't all that different after all.

Vignette 12: Kerrie

When Kerrie arrived at group for the sixth and final workshop, she was a little surprised to feel sad that group was ending. She remembered the first week, when she felt nervous and almost left before the workshop even started. Then, she remembered how relieved she was to learn that other parents in the group, and in her community, also had trans children. She thought about all the group meetings and the activities she had worked through; she thought about working on some of the activities with Dani and how happy he seemed when engaging with her through Chapter 4 and helping her identify what his needs might be as he transitions to adulthood. Kerrie realized that, through her work with the group, she felt seen and so did her son.

When group started, the leader congratulated all the participants for making it to week 6 of the program and told them that, this week, they would discuss advocacy – what it looks like and why it's important. Kerrie thoughtfully completed the activities and left room to add Dani's thoughts about how and with whom he would want his mom to advocate for him.

While working on the last activity in Chapter 6, "A Dream Revisited," Kerrie really felt herself come full circle from week one. She felt a little choked up as she recorded her current dream for Dani and realized that only the most important ideas from her first "Identity Dream" carried over: She dreamed for her son that he would be happy and healthy and surrounded by people who love and affirm him for who he is – an amazing young man. Kerrie planned in that moment to hang her new "dream" on the refrigerator when she got home so that she and Dani could remember to focus on what's really important in life, and that *that* has nothing to do with what other people think.

Reflection Questions

Image 6.8 A moment to reflect.

- As you look back over your journey through this workbook, what stands out to you the most?
- Did you experience a "light-bulb" moment, and if so, what was it?
- What have you learned about yourself that helps you affirm your LGBTQ+ teen?
- What new things have you learned about your teen as a result of engaging with this workbook?

References

Bronfenbrenner, U. (2000). Ecological systems theory. In A. E. Kazdin (Ed.), *Encyclopedia of psychology*, (Vol. 3). American Psychological Association. https://doi.org/10.1037/10518-046

Ceatha, N., Koay, A. C. C., Buggy, C., James, O., Tully, L., Bustillo, M., & Crowley, D. (2021). Protective factors for LGBTI+ youth wellbeing: A scoping review underpinned by recognition theory. *International Journal of Environmental Research and Public Health, 18*(21), 11682. https://doi.org/10.3390/ijerph182111682

Cottle, J., Drozdik, A. L., & Rimes, K. A. (2024). The impact of role models and mentors on the mental and physical wellbeing of sexual and gender minorities. *Behavioral Sciences, 14*(5), 417.

Earnest, M., Wong, S. L., Federico, S., & Cervantes, L. (2023). A model of advocacy to inform action. *Journal of General Internal Medicine, 38*(1), 208–212. https://doi.org/10.1007/s11606-022-07866-x

Ellard, K. K., Fairholme, C. P., Boisseau, C. L., Farchione, T. J., & Barlow, D. H. (2010). Unified protocol for the transdiagnostic treatment of emotional disorders: Protocol development and initial outcome data. *Cognitive and Behavioral Practice, 17*(1), 88–101. https://doi.org/10.1016/j.cbpra.2009.06.002

Epton, T., Currie, S., & Armitage, C. J. (2017). Unique effects of setting goals on behavior change: Systematic review and meta-analysis. *Journal of Consulting and Clinical Psychology, 85*(12), 1182–1198. https://doi.org/10.1037/ccp0000260

Knutson, D., Kertz, S., Chambers-Baltz, S., Christie, M., Harris, E., & Perinchery, R. (2020). A pilot test of a text message based transgender and non-binary affirmative cognitive behavioral intervention for anxiety and depression. Advance online publication. *Psychology of Sexual Orientation and Gender Diversity*. https://doi.org/10.1037/sgd0000438

Knutson, D., & Koch, J. M. (2018). Person-centered therapy as applied to work with transgender and gender-diverse clients. *Journal of Humanistic Psychology*. https://doi.org/10.1177/0022167818791082

Knutson, D., Matsuno, E., Goldbach, C., Hashtpari, H., & Smith, N. G. (2021). Advocating for transgender and non-binary affirmative spaces in graduate education. *Higher Education*. https://doi.org/10.1007/s10734-020-00673-5

Knutson, D., Soper, J., & Avance, R. (2025). Digital literacy for resistance: Implications for affirming practice with rural TNB youth and their families. *Journal of Health Service Psychology, 51*(2), 64–71.

Matsuno, E., & Israel, T. (2018). Psychological interventions promoting resilience among transgender individuals: Transgender resilience intervention model (TRIM). *The Counseling Psychologist, 46*(5), 632–655.

McConnell, E. A., Birkett, M., & Mustanski, B. (2016). Families matter: Social support and mental health trajectories among lesbian, gay, bisexual, and transgender youth. *Journal of Adolescent Health, 59*(6), 674–680. https://doi.org/10.1016/j.jadohealth.2016.07.026

McDonald, K. (2018). Social support and mental health in LGBTQ adolescents: A review of the literature. *Issues in Mental Health Nursing, 39*(1), 16–29.

McLaren, S., Bliss, L. R., Scott, C., Kraidler, P., & Pettignano, R. (2023). Applying a social ecological model to medical legal partnerships practice and research. *Journal of Law, Medicine & Ethics, 51*(4), 817–823. https://doi.org/10.1017/jme.2023.151

Milkman, R., Bloom, J., & Narro, V. (2010). *Working for justice: The L.A. model of organizing and advocacy.* Cornell University Press.

Miller, B., & Sprang, G. (2017). A components-based practice and supervision model for reducing compassion fatigue by affecting clinician experience. *Traumatology, 23*(2), 153–164. https://doi.org/10.1037/trm0000058

Murray, D. W., Rackers, H., Meyer, A., McKenzie, K. J., Malm, K., Sepulveda, K., & Heath, C. (2023). Co-regulation as a support for older youth in the context of foster care: A scoping review of the literature. *Prevention Science, 24*(6), 1187–1197.

Rabinowitz, Y. L., Yim, B., & Muran, J. C. (2025). Termination of psychotherapy: A systematic review. *Cogent Mental Health, 4*(1). https://doi.org/10.1080/28324765.2025.2535626

Springer, K. S., & Tolin, D. F. (2020). *The big book of exposures.* New Harbinger Publications.

Whittingham, K., & Coyne, L. W. (2019). Values and proto-values. In K. Whittingham, & L. W. Coyne (Eds.), *Acceptance and commitment therapy* (pp. 153–186). Academic Press.

Whittlesey, C. (2022). *The beginner's guide to being a trans ally.* Jessica Kingsley Publishers.

World Health Organization. (2023, December 1). *Human rights.* Author. https://www.who.int/news-room/fact-sheets/detail/human-rights-and-health

Yep, G. A. (2021). From being to doing: Toward a reconceptualization of LGBTQ worldmaking allies. *QED: A Journal in GLBTQ Worldmaking, 8*(2), 75–80. https://www.jstor.org/stable/48655678

APPENDIX A

ACTIVITY KEY AND RESOURCES

In this appendix, you will find answer keys that correspond with workbook activities. Some chapters will send you to this appendix to follow up on activities and exercises, but you are welcome to read over and revisit this section as needed. Feel free to use a highlighter or bookmark (both electronic and old-fashioned bookmarks will work) to save information you want to revisit later.

Activity 5 My Erasable Dictionary

Here are some possible definitions for the words listed in Activity 5:

Asexual: Describes individuals who do not experience sexual attraction.

Binary (i.e. Gender Binary): The idea that there are only two genders, male and female.

Bisexual: Describes an individual who has the capacity to form enduring physical, romantic, and/or emotional attractions to those of the same gender or to those of another gender.

Cis (as in Cisgender): Describes individuals whose gender identity is congruent with their sex assigned at birth.

Gay: Describes individuals whose enduring physical, romantic, and/or emotional attractions are to people of the same gender.

Gender Expression: The external ways a person communicates their gender, such as clothing, hair, mannerisms, activities, or social roles.

Gender Fluid: A term used to describe individuals whose gender changes over time.

Gender Identity: A person's deep internal sense of being female, male, or another identity.

Lesbian: A woman who has romantic and/or sexual orientation toward women.

Nonbinary: Describes individuals whose gender identity is not exclusively male or female. Individuals may identify as nonbinary or other identities, including but not limited to, genderqueer, agender, bigender, and genderfluid.

Pansexual: Describes individuals who experience sexual, romantic, physical, and/or spiritual attraction for members of all gender identities/expressions.

Queer: Historically, this has been a pejorative term used to describe LGBTQIA+ people, but is now used by some people, particularly younger people, whose sexual orientation is not exclusively straight/heterosexual. Some people may use queer, or more commonly genderqueer, to describe their gender identity and/or gender expression.

Questioning: A term used to describe individuals who are unsure about their sexual orientation and/or gender identity.

Sexual Orientation: A person's emotional, sexual, and/or relational attraction to others.

Trans: A shortened form of "transgender." Some people are starting to use the shortened form to acknowledge the identity piece that is not directly tied to gender.

Transgender: Describes individuals whose gender identity is different from the gender identity they were expected to have based on the sex they were assigned at birth.

Note: The definitions provided are based on commonly accepted understandings at the time of publication. These definitions are likely to change over time as noted in Chapter 2. We encourage you to research changes in these definitions frequently.

Activity 7 True or False

You can check your answers against the key, below. Boxes with an "X" through them contain incorrect information. Boxes that do not have an "X" through them contain correct information.

<table>
<tr><td>X LGBTQ+ people who get married do not stay together; the divorce rate is higher among LGBTQ+ couples.</td><td>The homelessness rate is higher among LGBTQ+ teens when compared to heterosexual, cis gender teens.</td><td>X Nonbinary people are diagnosed with autism at high rates because being nonbinary messes people up.</td><td>X Teens change their pronouns because it's a fad – it makes no difference in the long run what pronouns I use for my child.</td></tr>
<tr><td>X Most people who transition from one gender to another (e.g. male to female) end up regretting that decision.</td><td>X More LGBTQ+ teens identify as queer because it is popular, not because they really are LGBTQ+.</td><td>X Being LGBTQ+ is a choice some humans make; it's not natural.</td><td>LGBTQ+ teens are more likely to get addicted to drugs and alcohol.</td></tr>
<tr><td>LGBTQ+ teens are at a higher risk for suicide due to rejection and discrimination.</td><td>X It's not my place to correct someone if they use the wrong name or pronouns for my child.</td><td>Having just one affirming adult in their life can make a big difference in the mental health of an LGBTQ+ teen.</td><td>LGBTQ+ teens are highly resilient and able to counteract the impact of discrimination and oppression.</td></tr>
<tr><td>X Being gay or lesbian is just about sex.</td><td>X Polyamorous people just want to be promiscuous without any rules or standards.</td><td>X Being LGBTQ+ is completely incompatible with being a person of faith.</td><td>X I can have a strong relationship with my LGBTQ+ teen even though I do not accept their LGBTQ+ identity.</td></tr>
</table>

Activity 14 Identifying Myths and Facts

You can check your answers against the key, below. Boxes with an "X" through them contain incorrect information. Boxes that do not have an "X" through them contain correct information.

Girls who play with trucks when they are young grow up to be lesbians. (X)	LGBTQ+ teens cannot be Christian or join other communities of faith. (X)	Trans kids always tell their parents they are a different gender around age 3. (X)	LGBTQ+ teens are likely just going through a phase they will grow out of later. (X)
LGBTQ+ youth have a heightened risk of suicidal thoughts because they're confused about who they are. (X)	Boys who play with dolls at a young age are probably transgender. (X)	LGBTQ+ teens are highly resilient and able to live happy, fulfilled lives.	Boys grow up gay because their father was absent. (X)
As many as 11.6% of teens identify as LGBTQ+, indicating that it is not rare.	It's harmful to affirm young children who express an LGBTQ+ identity. (X)	LGBTQ+ teens and young adults who get married are more likely to divorce than other couples. (X)	Having just one affirming adult in their life can significantly reduce suicide risk for LGBTQ+ teens.
People who transition from one gender to another are incapable of having biological children. (X)	Most gay and/or trans men contract HIV/AIDS. (X)	LGBTQ+ kids are generally not affected by anti-LGBTQ+ legislation. (X)	Gay boys overidentify with or cling to their mothers and ultimately want to be women. (X)

Resource 1: Risk Awareness

As we stated elsewhere in this workbook, if you or your child is at immediate risk, you should call 911 or head to the nearest emergency room. The information in this section is not intended to replace professional care from a medical provider, behavioral health expert, or emergency response team. You can use this resource to build your awareness by helping you identify warning signs, risk factors, and protective factors. We offer a summary of risk indicators, but you can find more resources in the Bibliography in Appendix C (e.g., Baltazar, 2023; Liu & Mustanski, 2012). Please note that the lists that we provide are not exhaustive and we encourage you to look into other resources to learn more about suicide risk, self-harm, and other factors that impact children and youth.

Some Warning Signs

There are lots of warning signs that may signal increased risk. Individual warning signs are important to notice and address. The more warning signs a person shows, the more there may be cause for concern. Here are some warning signs to look out for:

- Isolation, depression, hopelessness, or worries about being a burden to others
- Low energy, loss of appetite, loss of interest in previously enjoyed activities
- Writing about, joking about, or even threatening suicide, death, or self-harm
- Preparing for death (such as by giving away items or writing "goodbye" notes)
- Engaging with media that involves death such as comics, movies, or internet searches
- Increases in aggression, anger, anxiety, or hostility
- Sudden calmness, resolve, or pronounced disinterest
- Sudden changes in behavior (such as impulsiveness, lack of self-care, or increased substance use)

Some Risk Factors

There are also lots of risk factors that can impact risk. Again, this is not a full list, but it is intended to give readers a place to start as they engage with the materials in this book. Some risk factors include:

- Previous attempt(s)
- Family dysfunction and distress
- Identification as LGBTQ+
- Chronic or major illness such as a cancer diagnosis, lupus, or a traumatic brain injury
- Psychiatric disorders such as bipolar disorder or a personality disorder
- High anxiety and post-traumatic stress disorders
- Substance use and impulsiveness
- Isolation and lack of social support
- Bullying

Some Protective Factors

The good news is that several things can help protect against risk. This entire workbook is designed to increase the quality of family relationships and decrease family distress (a major protective factor). Here is another (brief) list of some other protective factors:

- Optimism, hope, resilience, and a sense of purpose
- Access to nutrition and basic needs
- Access to medical, therapeutic, and support services
- Coping strategies and resources
- Community connections and social support
- Restricted (or no) access to substances, harmful media, and weapons

Resource 2: Calming Activities

There are lots of ways to regulate your emotions. We point out three common approaches that show up on a lot of websites, in books, and that are regularly used by therapists. Those common approaches are called a lot of things, but they basically boil down to intentional breathing and sensory grounding. Please note that grounding activities may distract you from distressing events (when they need your full attention) and not all activities work for everyone so they should be exercised with caution and intention. You might consider identifying calming activities that work for you with a therapist or other professional.

Intentional Breathing

One way to take a step back from a stressful situation is to shift your attention to your breathing. When you are stressed or feel threatened, your breathing usually speeds up, but breathing fast can actually contribute to your anxiety. When you shift attention to your breathing you stop focusing on your stress and you have a chance to start de-escalating your response. Intentionally slowing your breathing can really make a difference. Involving other parts of your body (such as using your finger to trace lines on a piece of paper) can help you refocus and level out even more. You will find a lot of diagrams and drawings you can trace while you slow your breathing, but we like using a rainbow (lots of authors, bloggers, and clinicians seem to feel the same). For the science behind breathing and stress, you can follow up on resources in the Bibliography in Appendix C (e.g., Hammond & Brown, 2025; Khng, 2023).

Sensory Grounding

Your senses (sight, touch, hearing, smell, and taste) can also provide you a way to refocus and calm yourself. Focusing on the world around you helps you ground yourself or locate yourself within your environment or present reality (when it is safe to shift or split your attention). Again, there are lots of diagrams and scripts you can use, scattered across the internet, and you can read more about them by following up on resources we included in our Bibliography in Appendix C (e.g., Hammond & Brown, 2025). The basic approach is to:

1. Name 5 things you see around you.
2. Name 4 things you can touch in your immediate vicinity.
3. Name 3 things you can hear.
4. Name 2 smells you can identify.
5. Name 1 thing you can taste.

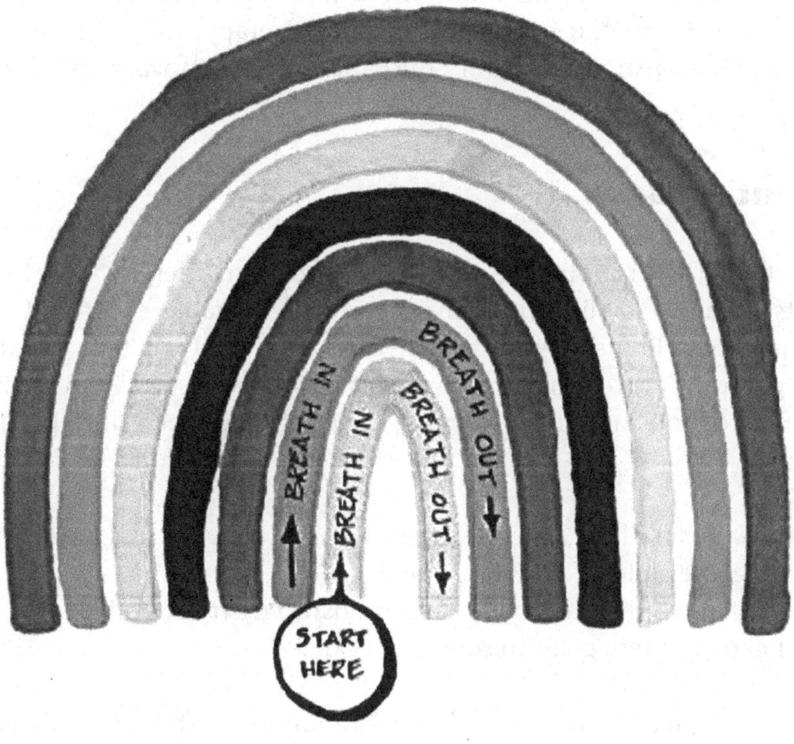

Image R.1 Breathing activity.

APPENDIX B

SCIENTIFIC BASES

Each step and activity is grounded in a scientific basis. When we wrote this workbook, we tried not to interrupt the flow of the chapters so that you could immerse yourself in the exercises and opportunities for self-reflection, but we still wanted you to be able to dig deeper into the science behind the work. In this section, we give you that chance to "look under the hood" of the workbook and further reflect on the content. This section is also written for group leaders and clinicians who may use this book in group settings or clinical practice. If you want to follow up on the resources cited via in-text citations, you can find the reference resources used in this section listed in the bibliography.

Activity 1: Scientific Basis

Scholars note that the imagination can be an important tool used to process challenges, think through uncomfortable situations, and reduce distress (Singer & Pope, 2012). Solution-focused therapists sometimes use the "magic wand" question that allows clients to think about what life would be like if their problems were solved and they were living the way they wanted to (Wells & McCaig, 2016). This exercise is designed to help you reflect on how you thought, felt, and behaved when your child came out to you as LGBTQ+. Similar to solution-focused therapy, this exercise helped you examine where you are in your relationship with your child and where you want to go as you work through this workbook.

Activity 2: Scientific Basis

If you have ever participated in individual or group, outpatient therapy, you know how important goals are. Therapists usually establish clear, measurable, achievable goals that guide the therapeutic process and ensure that clients stay on track (Matre et al., 2013). This workbook leverages that goal-setting tool to guide you through the activities that follow. If you want to optimize your use of the workbook, feel free to look back at the learning contract you filled out in Chapter 1 and ask yourself questions like:

- How will I know when I have reached these goals?
- Are these goals achievable in a 6-week period?
- How will the goals help me improve my relationship with my child?
- How would I explain these goals to someone else?

If you want, you can jot down an answer to each question underneath it or on a separate sheet of paper.

Activity 3: Scientific Basis

Many parents go through a period of adjustment when their child discloses their LGBTQ+ identity that can include a grief process, denial, and other distress-driven experiences (e.g., D'amico et al., 2015). These difficulties can cause a lot of guilt, pain, and regret. The data we have collected from parenting groups indicates that parents benefit from taking their experiences at face value, in a nonjudgmental space, where they are able to both challenge and accept their reactions. In other words, parents grow when they challenge their own conditions of worth and "shoulds," consistent with person-centered approaches to therapy (Rogers et al., 2022).

Activity 4: Scientific Basis

Therapists have varying feelings about safety plans and their effectiveness, but researchers suggest that they are generally effective at reducing risk, especially among highly distressed populations (Ferguson et al., 2021). There is further evidence that the benefits of safety planning extend to digital, online, self-guided formats (Rainbow et al., 2024). In any case, safety plans tend to be more effective when they are personalized, perceived as useful, and person-centered. We encourage readers to invest in the safety planning process as an act of self-care and to see the process as an opportunity to engage in self-love rather than just a task to be completed.

Activity 5: Scientific Basis

There is a lot of evidence that including pronouns is an essential part of supporting LGBTQ+ people and identity related language is a key part of clinical treatment (e.g., Knutson et al., 2019). The fact that terminology changes is a clear marker of its psychological importance, not an indicator that LGBTQ+ people are being tricky, indecisive, or disingenuous (Galupo et al., 2017). Scholars who research gender dysphoria and other forms of distress suggest that creating affirming environments makes a huge difference and distress that shows up outwardly (e.g., depression, anxiety) may be markers of the impact of the environment (Goldbach & Knutson, 2021). Work with identity-based language is not tangential to LGBTQ+-affirming care, it is central to the work.

Activity 6: Scientific Basis

Clinical scientists note that maladaptive coping skills provide relief from distress and that demanding patients discontinue maladaptive behaviors immediately (instead of working through risk reduction strategies) can increase the risk of more extreme coping strategies (see Rogers et al., 2022). Of course, baggage related to having an LGBTQ+ child is not remotely similar to self-harm, but the intensity of emotion surrounding a child's LGBTQ+ identity can be pretty intense (Holodynski & Kärtner, 2023). When we have administered this workbook in groups, parents have talked about social pressures and messages telling them to 'just get over it.' That message can be very counterproductive, especially in clinical spaces. Building parental self-efficacy involves identifying strengths and helping parents to grow by expanding their strengths, not confronting them with their growth edges (Jefferson et al., 2020).

Activity 7: Scientific Basis

A core principle of Cognitive Behavioral Therapy (Beck, 1964) is that core beliefs shape behaviors, thoughts and feelings. In other words, what we believe matters. For example, misinformation about LGBTQ+ people can be weaponized and used to shape political views and voting behaviors (Knutson et al., 2021). Therefore, it is not only important to equip families with affirming skills, it is also important to examine beliefs that may help or hinder them from using those skills. You may be familiar with the Stages of Change model (Prochaska & DiClemente, 1983) and the idea that knowing about an issue is not the only step toward changing it. Parents and guardians may spend a lot of time in pre-contemplation and contemplation stages before moving toward positive change in their families. Challenging closely held beliefs can be hard work, but it is an essential part of setting families up for success because it can help them move into action.

Activity 8: Scientific Basis

There have been a lot of arguments over what kind of therapy works the best. Researchers and scholars can argue endlessly about whether, for example, Cognitive Behavioral Therapies are the most effective way to treat most behavioral health concerns. However, there is some evidence that most therapeutic approaches share common elements that make them effective (Rosenzweig, 1936). To put it a different way, most therapies are effective for the same reasons. This is called the Dodo bird hypothesis or the Dodo bird verdict, a reference to the Dodo bird in Lewis Carroll's (1865) Alice's Adventures in Wonderland who declares everyone a winner (Rosenzweig, 1936). We suggest that this is also true about relationship-building with teens. There are a lot of ways to build relationships (e.g., playing sports together, going to movies, reading the same book), but healthy relationships in families and approaches to building them have common factors like empathy, dedication, and shared goals. In this chapter, we emphasized a common factor that is important in therapeutic and family relationships alike: trust.

Activity 9: Scientific Basis

The World Professional Association for Transgender Health (WPATH) maintains standards of care for gender-affirming care that have been revised over the years and the most recent edition is version 8 (Coleman et al., 2022). A core idea behind the WPATH approach to trans and nonbinary identities (and by extension, other LGBTQ+ identities) is that queer identity is three dimensional and may include infinite possibilities. That view is consistent with identity development models that frame gender and sexual orientation development as a process that plays out across the lifespan (e.g., Bilodeau & Renn, 2005). The point is that there is no "right" destination when it comes to gender identity and sexual orientation. Healing comes when people are seen for who they are and their journey toward discovering themselves is affirmed. That goes for parents and teens alike.

Activity 10: Scientific Basis

Before parents try to understand the identities of their teens, it is important for them to understand their own identities. It is much easier for a person to be interested (and not just curious) in other people when they know themselves, their own perspectives, and their own beliefs (Lind & Thomsen, 2018; Thomsen & Pillemer, 2017). This is one of the reasons that behavioral health training programs help trainees face their biases, explore their own needs, and engage with people who are different or cultures that are unfamiliar (e.g., Ratts et al., 2016). Just like therapists, parents are more likely to stay calm, focused, and helpful when they have thought through their own experiences and prepared to help others from a firm foundation of self-understanding.

Activity 11: Scientific Basis

This exercise is a concrete way for parents, guardians, and even teens to explore gender role dynamics, a core theme in feminist therapeutic approaches (Corey & Herlihy, 2012). Feminist and multicultural therapists have long pointed out that deviating from societal expectations can open people up to rejection, discrimination, and violence, but they have also pointed out that conforming to restrictive societal expectations can cause distress for everyone, even the people who benefit from those norms (e.g., American Psychological Association, Boys and Men Guidelines Group, 2018. APA guidelines for psychological practice with boys and men. American Psychological Association, Boys and Men Guidelines Group, 2018). Parents may benefit from not only exploring ways they get punished for deviating from societal expectations, but they may also gain a lot from exploring what they give up in order to meet societal standards, especially when those standards are arbitrary or unnecessary.

Activity 12: Scientific Basis

Identifying emotions is hard and it takes a lot of practice (Tsvieli et al., 2020). Sometimes we encourage therapists in training to pair this emotion iceberg exercise with a feelings word list or feelings wheel that helps clients identify and verbalize emotions that they are less familiar with. Building an emotional vocabulary can take time, even for therapists. This activity takes a lot of self-compassion. Parents should be reminded that "getting good" at sharing feelings does not happen overnight. However, the very act of trying to share emotions (especially when they are received and validated) can help families heal. It is important to remember that having just one supportive adult reduces the suicide risk in LGBTQ+ teens (Nath et al., 2025). Effectively sharing and engaging with emotions is hard work, but it pays off.

Activity 13: Scientific Basis

Researchers and scholars have spent a lot of time trying to figure out what "makes" LGBTQ+ youth turn out to be LGBTQ+ (Lewis & Reynolds, 2025). The reality is that there is no single factor or characteristic that sets LGBTQ+ youth apart (LeVay, 2016). No matter how hard they have tried, scientists have been unable to locate a gene, parenting behavior, developmental milestone, or chemical in the water that makes a person LGBTQ+ (Satinover, 1996). For example, some gay boys love football and others do not. The way a person grew up relating to football has nothing to do with their identity. Knowing that may help parents, but there is an even more important and healthy insight from the current data that parents need to be aware of: There is nothing you can do or un-do to change your child's identity (American Psychological Association, 2009). In fact, trying to shape a child's gender or sexual orientation can actually cause distress and trauma. Parents bear witness to their teen's development and every moment (the year they try out bangs, refuse to wear off-brand clothes, and so on) is an opportunity to marvel and embrace the memories.

Activity 14: Scientific Basis

In Chapter 2, following the myth and fact activity, we talked about how beliefs shape behaviors, thoughts and feelings (Beck, 1976). That is important to consider when reflecting on the impact misinformation can have on your relationship with your LGBTQ+ teen and it is relevant to this exercise as well. Beliefs about development can have another impact, though, that we started discussing in this section. When parents believe there is something wrong with being LGBTQ+, they can start looking for evidence to support that belief. Looking for evidence to support a preexisting belief is called "confirmation bias" (Oswald & Grosjean, 2004). For example, if you believe you are a loser and people do not like you and then you see a group of people laughing at the grocery store, you might think, "See, they think I am a loser and they are laughing at me." Confirmation bias can make people more susceptible to believing false information, even when it does not make a lot of sense (Oswald & Grosjean, 2004). Not only is it important for parents to push back against confirmation biases that frame their teen as sick or disordered simply because they are LGBTQ+, it can also open up opportunities for empathy. Parents can probably identify a time their teen made assumptions based on a belief that people do not like them even when it did not make sense. Identifying and pushing back on things like confirmation bias can help parents see and challenge those unhelpful beliefs in their teens as well.

Activity 15: Scientific Basis

In today's society, misinformation can run rampant (Aïmeur et al., 2023). With the rise of AI and the increasing sophistication of search engines (that do not just find websites, but also try to give you answers), it can be hard to distinguish between what is real and reliable and what is not. That kind of uncertainty can cause psychological stress (Levine et al., 1975) and times of crisis can make finding information even harder to navigate (Bursztyn et al., 2020). We believe parents are more likely to maintain a feeling of confidence and address crises when they establish consistent sources of information and support well in advance of needing it. That way, they know where to turn when they face a challenge or are asked a question for which they do not have a ready answer. Different sources of information can meet different needs, and that awareness can help parents resist over relying on their LGBTQ+ teen for insights and support. That, in turn, can help remove some of the pressure and stress from LGBTQ+ teens who are already facing a lot of uncertainty and pressure.

Activity 16: Scientific Basis

Researchers have studied LGBTQ+ youth in the transitional stage between adolescence and adulthood and identified a variety of risk factors that are associated with increases in vulnerability and negative health behaviors (e.g., Knutson et al., 2021). When youth transition out of their childhood homes and take on a greater level of independence, parents may feel as if they have less control or influence over their behaviors, safety, and well-being. That may be the case, but parents can draw a lot of solace from knowing they did their best and set their child up for success. Starting that process well before the transitional phase helps instill in parents a sort of mindfulness or awareness of the process and a sense that they have an influence on the outcome. In general, mindfulness and awareness are key components of psychological health and healing processes (Keng et al., 2011).

Activity 17: Scientific Basis

When we collected focus group data on this workbook, several stakeholders (e.g., teachers, parents, and researchers) encouraged us to remind parents to involve their teens in key decisions related to the coming out process. They were pointing out something very important about the psychological and interpersonal impacts of being "outed" or having private information shared with others without consent. Researchers found that forced disclosure or "being outed" to parents, for example, is associated with depressive symptoms and reduced parental support (McCauley et al., 2024). It probably is not hard for parents and guardians to empathize with this experience, especially if they reflect on times they told someone a secret and then discovered their secret had been shared. There is a growing body of research exploring the complex dynamics, interpersonal implications, and emotional responses to secret sharing that further reinforce the impact disclosures or "outing" can have on key, close relationships (e.g., Bedrov & Gable, 2023).

Activity 18: Scientific Basis

Researchers and scholars have extensively discussed barriers to LGBTQ+-affirming health services both broadly and in specific situations such as in rural and remote areas (e.g., Koch & Knutson, 2016). As we noted earlier in this workbook, it is important not to lose sight of the incredible resilience that LGBTQ+ people possess (e.g., Matsuno & Israel, 2018), but it is also important for parents to prepare for the challenges and barriers to care they are likely to face. When working with parents of LGBTQ+ teens, it may be helpful to take a "hope for the best, prepare for the worst" approach. In addition to this workbook, scholars are developing a wide range of resources to support parents (e.g., Matsuno & Israel, 2021), and researchers are even developing guides (such as the Digital Literacy for Resistance approach) for providers who work with parents of LGBTQ+ youth to assist them with responding to crises and social pressures (e.g., Knutson et al., 2025).

Activity 19: Scientific Basis

This activity was added after we started piloting this workbook with parents and guardians of LGBTQ+ youth in a rural-facing clinic. Exasperated parents kept sharing stories about times their teens "freaked out" in ways that did not make sense to the parents. The parents would share things like, "I just told my teen that they had to get out of the house and walk to the park with me and they started bawling." We added this section to help parents make sense of the heightened emotional states they may observe in their LGBTQ+ teens and to do so, we drew on neuroscientific research such as discussions of the "Hand Model of the Brain" (Siegel & Payne Bryson, 2011). When teens get dysregulated, parents can feel pressure to "double down" or discipline their youth (or they can become dysregulated themselves), but they are unlikely to succeed at getting through to their teen if the teen has entered a state of dysregulation and fear of rejection related to their LGBTQ+ identity. Therapists and support providers may benefit from helping parents identify signs of dysregulation so they can respond by increasing their teen's sense of safety before addressing the core issues.

Activity 20: Scientific Basis

The SHELL model is used in aviation (Hawkins, 1987), but to our knowledge the acronym has not been applied to parenting (in aviation safety circles the words in our acronym stand for different concepts). In any case, the parenting SHELL model rests on a foundation of empathy. That is to say that identifying the reason for dysregulation is important because it builds empathy (Zaki, 2020). When teens are dysregulated, it is not usually because they are trying to be difficult (they want connection, not disconnection). When an infant cries, parents usually try to draw inferences (they must be hungry, cold, thirsty, etc.), and they try to meet those needs, but somehow that impulse gets lost when children grow into teenagers. It is easy to forget that emotional outbursts can be indicators of unmet needs. Behaviorists would suggest that all behavior has meaning (Maze, 2019), and in the case of emotional crises, teens are often looking for a way out of distress. Helping parents refocus on the meaning behind a behavior, rather than taking it at face value, is one way to strengthen family bonds especially for LGBTQ+ youth who face daily rejection, discrimination, and stressors that can increase emotional reactivity and a need for safe spaces.

Activity 21: Scientific Basis

As we have indicated throughout this book, parents are a key source of support for LGBTQ+ teens (Ceatha et al., 2021; McConnell et al., 2016). When parents show up for their teens and refuse to give in to the "powers that be," they give their teens a better chance at life. However, this process does not occur in a vacuum. As we noted in the precursor to the worksheet, parents should collaborate with teens (as appropriate) to construct their advocacy plans. Involving teens in that process ensures parents are (a) advocating with the consent and buy-in of their teens, (b) meeting the actual needs of their teens, and (c) teaching their teen how to advocate for themself. Role models can have a big, positive impact on LGBTQ+ teens (Cottle et al., 2024), and parents can be some of the most powerful role models of all. The more parents dare to dream big, the more they create a world in which their teen's dreams can come true. Parents may benefit from regular encouragement to keep dreaming, to never stop believing that positive change is possible.

Activity 22: Scientific Basis

Researchers who work with LGBTQ+ communities have been placing greater and greater emphasis on the role of resilience in LGBTQ+ health (e.g., Matsuno & Israel, 2018). Interventions intended to increase resilience, reduce distress, and expand social support for LGBTQ+ people prioritize a number of strategies to increase health that target avoidance, facilitate the expression of needs, and encourage participation in activism (Knutson et al., 2020; Matsuno & Israel, 2018). Parents of LGBTQ+ youth can use similar strategies as advocates for their teens. As we discussed earlier, modeling is an important component of advocacy. In fact, when parents model advocacy for their teens, they engage in many of the resilience strategies that have been identified by researchers as key to LGBTQ+ resilience such as positive role modeling, acceptance, social support, and family acceptance (Matsuno & Israel, 2018). Working through resistance or approaching sources of fear may seem like a simple skill, but in the context of parenting LGBTQ+ teens, it is a transformative act that can encourage change at multiple ecological levels.

Activity 23: Scientific Basis

As we have discussed elsewhere in this book, we take a person-centered, humanistic approach to parenting LGBTQ+ youth that recognizes the central role of relationships in the health and resilience of LGBTQ+ people (see Knutson & Koch, 2018). One of the consistent themes that came up as we designed and piloted this workbook was the need for social support and social connections shared by parents of LGBTQ+ youth, especially those located in rural and remote areas. That is one of the reasons we opened and concluded this book with an acknowledgement that parents of LGBTQ+ teens are not alone. Clinicians may benefit from reinforcing that truth and by using the materials in this workbook to facilitate connections between parents both within and outside of clinical spaces. Parenting is a tough job under any circumstances, but it gets a little easier when parents do not have to do it alone.

Activity 24: Scientific Basis

Termination or the end of a therapeutic relationship can be hard, complex, and even messy (Rabinowitz et al., 2025). Reasons for termination can vary from mutual to forced or premature. Likewise, the impact of termination can impact therapists and clients in different ways. The reality is that terminations just are not easy. However, we believe that terminations can also be healing, supportive, and empowering. Toward that end, this workbook is designed to, in some sense, refer parents to themselves for ongoing care. In other words, parents are invited to reconnect with themselves, their dreams, and their futures. They are encouraged to continue the discovery they started and maintain confidence that they are equal to the task of parenting an LGBTQ+ teen. Therapists who use this workbook may benefit from emphasizing empowerment, self-determination, and self-efficacy as they guide parenting groups and individual clients through the end of this workbook. As with any termination, it may be helpful for participants to remember that they can always come back to therapy for support and needing help is not failure. Asking for help is a strength.

APPENDIX C

BIBLIOGRAPHY

This appendix includes a list of the works cited in the chapters, scientific bases (Appendix B), and helpful resources. Readers can use this appendix as a source of additional readings or can dig deeper into important research that was used to create this workbook. It is impossible to provide an exhaustive list of all of the important work related to LGBTQ+ youth, but this list contains many of the major resources parents and clinicians may find helpful.

Resources

Abreu, R. L., Gonzalez, K. A., Rosario, C. C., Pulice-Farrow, L., & Rodríguez, M. M. D. (2020). "Latinos have a stronger attachment to the family": Latinx fathers' acceptance of their sexual minority children. *Journal of GLBT Family Studies, 16*(2), 192–210. https://doi.org/10.1080/1550428X.2019.1672232

Abreu, R. L., Martin, J. A., & Badio, K. S. (2023). Latinx LGBTQ people and their families: The role of Latinx cultural values, beliefs, and traditions. In J. M. Koch, E. E. Townsend-Bell, & R. D. Hubach (Eds.), *Identity as resilience in minoritized communities: Strengths-based approaches to research and practice* (pp. 47–58). Springer Nature Switzerland. https://doi.org/10.1007/978-3-031-38977-1_4

Abreu, R. L., McEachern, A. G., & Kenny, M. C. (2017). Myths and misconceptions about LGBTQ Youth: School counselors' role in advocacy. *Journal of School Counseling, 15*(8). https://eric.ed.gov/?id=EJ1146191

Acton, G. J. (2002). Health-promoting self-care in family caregivers. *Western Journal of Nursing Research, 24*(1), 73–86.

Aïmeur, E., Amri, S., & Brassard, G. (2023). Fake news, disinformation and misinformation in social media: A review. *Social Network Analysis and Mining, 13*(1), 30.

American Academy of Child & Adolescent Psychiatry. (2018). *Conversion therapy.* https://www.aacap.org/aacap/Policy_Statements/2018/Conversion_Therapy.aspx

American Counseling Association. (2014). *2014 ACA code of ethics.* https://www.counseling.org/docs/default-source/default-document-library/ethics/2014-aca-code-of-ethics.pdf

American Medical Association. (2022). *Advocating for the LGBTQ community.* https://www.ama-assn.org/delivering-care/population-care/advocating-lgbtq-community

American Psychological Association. (2009). *Report of the American Psychological Association task force on appropriate affirmative responses to sexual orientation.* https://www.apa.org/pi/lgbt/resources/therapeutic-response.pdf

American Psychological Association, Boys and Men Guidelines Group. (2018). *APA guidelines for psychological practice with boys and men.* http://www.apa.org/about/policy/psychological-practice-boys-men-guidelines.pdf

Arnett, J. J. (2004). *Emerging adulthood: The winding road from the late teens through the twenties.* Oxford University Press.

Balmores-Paulino, R. S. (2020). Avoidance coping strategies. In V. Zeigler-Hill, & T. K. Shackelford (Eds.), *Encyclopedia of personality and individual differences* (pp. 343–344). Springer International Publishing.

Baltazar, A. (2023). Self-harm: Warning signs, risk factors, and prevention. *Journal of Family Research and Practice, 3*(1), 13. https://www.nadfamily.org/resources/journal/

Bandura, A. (1977). *Social learning theory*. Prentice-Hall.

Beck, A. T. (1976). *Cognitive therapy and the emotional disorders*. International Universities Press.

Bedrov, A., & Gable, S. L. (2023). Just between us . . .: The role of sharing and receiving secrets in friendship across time. *Personal Relationships, 31*(1), 91–111. https://doi.org/10.1111/pere.12527

Bilodeau, B., & Renn, K. A. (2005). Analysis of LGBT identity development models and implications for practice. *New Directions for Student Services*, 25–39.

Birnkrant, J. M., & and Przeworski, A. (2017). Communication, advocacy, and acceptance among support-seeking parents of transgender youth. *Journal of Gay & Lesbian Mental Health, 21*(2), 132–153. https://doi.org/10.1080/19359705.2016.1277173

Bronfenbrenner, U. (2000). Ecological systems theory. In A. E. Kazdin (Ed.) *Encyclopedia of psychology*, (Vol. 3). American Psychological Association. https://doi.org/10.1037/10518-046

Brown, B. (2012). *Daring greatly: How the courage to be vulnerable transforms the way we live, love, parent, and lead.* Penguin Random House.

Brown, C., Porta, C. M., Eisenberg, M. E., McMorris, B. J., & Sieving, R. E. (2020). Family relationships and the health and well-being of transgender and gender-diverse youth: A critical review. *LGBT Health, 7*(8), 407–419. https://doi.org/10.1089/lgbt.2019.0200

Bull, B., & D'Arrigo-Patrick, J. (2018). Parent experiences of a child's social transition: Moving beyond the loss narrative. *Journal of Feminist Family Therapy, 30*(3), 170–190. https://doi.org/10.1080/08952833.2018.1448965

Bursztyn, L., Rao, A., Roth, C. P., & Yanagizawa-Drott, D. H. (2020). *Misinformation during a pandemic* (No. w27417). National Bureau of Economic Research.

Campbell, D. G., Guimarães, J. A. C., Pinho, F. A., Martínez-Ávila, D., & Nascimento, F. A. (2017). The terminological polyhedron in LGBTQ terminology: Self-naming as a power to empower in knowledge organization. *Knowledge Organization, 44*(8), 586–591. https://doi.org/10.5771/0943-7444-2017-8-586

Campbell, S. B., & Renshaw, K. D. (2018). Posttraumatic stress disorder and relationship functioning: A comprehensive review and organizational framework. *Clinical Psychology Review, 65*, 152–162. https://doi.org/10.1016/j.cpr.2018.08.003

Carroll, L. (1865). *Alice's adventures in Wonderland*. Macmillan Publishers.

Ceatha, N., Koay, A. C. C., Buggy, C., James, O., Tully, L., Bustillo, M., & Crowley, D. (2021). Protective factors for LGBTI+ youth wellbeing: A scoping review underpinned by recognition theory. *International Journal of Environmental Research and Public Health, 18*(21), 11682. https://doi.org/10.3390/ijerph182111682

Coleman, E., Radix, A. E., Bouman, W. P., Brown, G. R., de Vries, A. L. C., Deutsch, M. B., . . . Arcelus, J. (2022). Standards of care for the health of transgender and gender diverse people, version 8. *International Journal of Transgender Health, 23*(sup1), S1–S259. https://doi.org/10.1080/26895269.2022.2100644

Corey, G., & Herlihy, B. (2012). Chapter 12: Feminist theory. In G. Corey (Ed.), *Theory and practice of counseling and psychotherapy* (9th ed., pp. 360–394). CENGAGE Learning Custom Publishing. https://nibmehub.com/opacservice/pdf/read/Theory%20and%20Practice%20of%20Counseling%20and%20Psychotherapy-%20Corey-%209ed.pdf

Cramer, R. J., Golom, F. D., LoPresto, C. T., & Kirkley, S. M. (2008). Weighing the evidence: Empirical assessment and ethical implications of conversion therapy. *Ethics & Behavior, 18*(1), 93–114. https://doi.org/10.1080/10508420701713014

D'amico, E., Julien, D., Tremblay, N., & Chartrand, E. (2015). Gay, lesbian, and bisexual youths coming out to their parents: Parental reactions and youths' outcomes. *Journal of GLBT Family Studies, 11*(5), 411–437. https://doi.org/10.1080/1550428X.2014.981627

DeChants, J. P., Shelton, J., Anyon, Y., & Bender, K. (2022). "It kinda breaks my heart": LGBTQ young adults' responses to family rejection. *Family Relations, 71*(3), 968–986. https://doi.org/10.1111/fare.12638

Denes, A., & Afifi, T. D. (2014). Coming out again: Exploring GLBQ individuals' communication with their parents after the first coming out. *Journal of GLBT Family Studies, 10*(3), 298–325. https://doi.org/10.1080/1550428X.2013.838150

Earnest, M., Wong, S. L., Federico, S., & Cervantes, L. (2023). A model of advocacy to inform action. *Journal of General Internal Medicine, 38*(1), 208–212. https://doi.org/10.1007/s11606-022-07866-x

Egan, J. D., Tolman, S., McBrayer, J. S., & Ballesteros, E. (2023). Reconceptualizing Kolb's learning cycle as episodic & lifelong. *Experiential Learning and Teaching in Higher Education, 6*(1), 24–33. https://doi.org/10.46787/elthe.v6i1.3607

Egolf, A., & Gold, A. L. (2023). Interpersonal effectiveness in action: The therapeutic milieu for DBT assertiveness skills practice. *Brown University Child & Adolescent Behavior Letter, 39*(3), 1–4. https://doi.org/10.1002/cbl.30693

Ellard, K. K., Fairholme, C. P., Boisseau, C. L., Farchione, T. J., & Barlow, D. H. (2010). Unified protocol for the transdiagnostic treatment of emotional disorders: Protocol development and initial outcome data. *Cognitive and Behavioral Practice, 17*(1), 88–101. https://doi.org/10.1016/j.cbpra.2009.06.002

Epton, T., Currie, S., & Armitage, C. J. (2017). Unique effects of setting goals on behavior change: Systematic review and meta-analysis. *Journal of Consulting and Clinical Psychology, 85*(12), 1182–1198. https://doi.org/10.1037/ccp0000260

Ferguson, M., Rhodes, K., Loughhead, M., McIntyre, H., & Procter, N. (2021). The effectiveness of the safety planning intervention for adults experiencing suicide-related distress: A systematic review. *Archives of Suicide Research, 26*(3), 1022–1045. https://doi.org/10.1080/13811118.2021.1915217

Galupo, M. P., Pulice-Farrow, L., & Ramirez, J. L. (2017). "Like a constantly flowing river": Gender identity flexibility among nonbinary transgender individuals. In J. Sinnott (Ed.), *Identity flexibility during adulthood*. Cham: Springer. https://doi.org/10.1007/978-3-319-55658-1_10

Garofalo, R. (2023). Editor's Statement: Using misinformation to harm LGBTQ people is not new. *Transgender Health, 8*(4), 300–301. https://doi.org/10.1089/trgh.2023.29001.editorial

Goldbach, C., & Knutson, D. (2021, November 29). Gender-related minority stress and gender dysphoria: Development and initial validation of the Gender Dysphoria Triggers Scale (GDTS). *Psychology of Sexual Orientation and Gender Diversity*. Advance online publication. http://dx.doi.org/10.1037/sgd0000548

González-González, F., Strizzi, J. M., & Fernández-Agis, I. (2025). "Accepting a transgender child is to improve the way one lives on this planet": Support and acceptance trajectories of parents of transgender and gender diverse children. *LGBTQ+ Family: An Interdisciplinary Journal, 21*(2), 101–115. https://doi.org/10.1080/27703371.2024.2370883

Goodman, L. A., Wilson, J. M., Helms, J. E., Greenstein, N., & Medzhitova, J. (2018). Becoming an advocate: Processes and outcomes of a relationship-centered advocacy training model. *The Counseling Psychologist, 46*(2), 122–153. https://doi.org/10.1177/0011000018757168

Gorse, M. (2022). Risk and protective factors to LGBTQ+ youth suicide: A review of the literature. *Child and Adolescent Social Work Journal, 39*(1), 17–28. https://doi.org/10.1007/s10560-020-00710-3

Gray, S. A. O., Sweeney, K. K., Randazzo, R., & Levitt, H. M. (2016). "Am I doing the right thing?": Pathways to parenting a gender variant child. *Family Process, 55*(1), 123–138. https://doi.org/10.1111/famp.12128

Greenfield, J. (2008). Coming out: The process of forming a positive identity. In H. J. Makadon, & J. Potter (Eds.), *The Fenway guide to lesbian, gay, bisexual, and transgender health* (pp. 45–74). ACP Press.

Grossmann, I., Peetz, J., Dorfman, A., Rotella, A., & Buehler, R. (2024). The wise mind balances the abstract and the concrete. *Open Mind: Discoveries in Cognitive Science, 8*, 826–858. https://doi.org/10.1162/opmi_a_00149

Guest, L. M. H., & Weinstein, N. (2020). The effect of healthcare provider support and discrimination on LGBT patients' trust and adherence. *The British Student Doctor Journal, 4*(3), 37–39. https://doi.org/10.18573/bsdj.204

Hadland, S. E., Yehia, B. R., & Makadon, H. J. (2016). Caring for lesbian, gay, bisexual, transgender, and questioning youth in inclusive and affirmative environments. *Pediatric Clinics, 63*(6), 955–969. https://doi.org/10.1016/j.pcl.2016.07.001

Hafeez, H., Zeshan, M., Tahir, M. A., Jahan, N., Naveed, S., Hafeez, H., Zeshan, M., Tahir, M. A., Jahan, N., & Naveed, S. (2017). Health care disparities among lesbian, gay, bisexual, and transgender youth: A literature review. *Cureus, 9*(4). https://doi.org/10.7759/cureus.1184

Haines, E. L., Deaux, K., & Lofaro, N. (2016). The times they are a-changing . . . or are they not? A comparison of gender stereotypes, 1983–2014. *Psychology of Women Quarterly, 40*(3), 353–363.

Haldeman, D. C. (2022). *The case against conversion "therapy": Evidence, ethics, and alternatives*. American Psychological Association.

Hammond, J., & Brown, W. J. (2025). Building an operational definition of grounding. *Trauma, Violence, & Abuse*. https://doi.org/10.1177/15248380251343189

Hawkins, F. H. (1987). *Human factors in flight*. Gower Technical Press.

Hawkins, J. D., Smith, B. H., & Catalano, R. F. (2004). Social development and social and emotional learning. In J. E. Zins, R. P. Weissberg, M. C. Wang, & H. J. Walberg (Eds.), *Building academic success on social and emotional learning: What does the research say?* (pp. 135–150). Teachers College Press.

Holodynski, M., & Kärtner, J. (2023). Parental coregulation of child emotions. In I. Roskam, J. J. Gross, & M. Mikolajczak (Eds.), *Emotion regulation and parenting* (pp. 129–148). Cambridge University Press.

Imaz-Sheinbaum, M. (2021). Principles of narrative reason. *History & Theory*, *60*(2), 249–270. https://doi.org/10.1111/hith.12205

Jefferson, F. A., Shires, A., & McAloon, J. (2020). Parenting self-compassion: A systematic review and meta-analysis. *Mindfulness*, *11*(9), 2067–2088. https://doi.org/10.1007/s12671-020-01401-x

Johnson, K. C., LeBlanc, A. J., Sterzing, P. R., Deardorff, J., Antin, T., & Bockting, W. O. (2020). Trans adolescents' perceptions and experiences of their parents' supportive and rejecting behaviors. *Journal of Counseling Psychology*, *67*(2), 156–170. https://doi.org/10.1037/cou0000419

Kayman, D. J., Goldstein, M. F., Dixon, L., & Goodman, M. (2015). Perspectives of suicidal veterans on safety planning. *Crisis*, *36*(5), 371–383. https://doi.org/10.1027/0227-5910/a000348

Keng, S. L., Smoski, M. J., & Robins, C. J. (2011). Effects of mindfulness on psychological health: A review of empirical studies. *Clinical Psychology Review*, *31*(6), 1041–1056.

Kennedy, A. (2024). Intersex. In *Salem Press Encyclopedia*. Salem Press.

Khng, K. H. (2023). Deep breathing and mindfulness: Simple techniques to promote students' self-regulation and well-being from the inside out. In R. B. King, I. S. Caleon, & A. B. I. Bernardo (Eds.), *Positive psychology and positive education in Asia*. Singapore: Springer. https://doi.org/10.1007/978-981-99-5571-8_17

Knutson, D., Goldbach, C., & Koch, J. (2022). *Counseling in a gender expansive world: Resources to support therapeutic practice*. Rowman & Littlefield.

Knutson, D., Jacobs, S. C., Hakman, M., & Milton, D. C. (2021). Profiles of distress and self-harm among LGBTQ+ transitional youth in a rural state. *Journal of Rural Mental Health*, *45*(2), 107–120. https://doi.org/10.1037/rmh0000168

Knutson, D., Koch, J. M., & Goldbach, C. (2019). Recommended terminology, pronouns, and documentation for work with transgender and non-binary populations. *Practice Innovations*, *4*(4), 214–224. https://doi.org/10.1037/pri0000098

Knutson, D., Peter-Hagene, C., & Satveer, K. (2021). Liberal political orientation strengthens the positive relationship between religiosity and bathroom bill support. *Sexuality Research and Public Policy*. https://doi.org/10.1007/s13178-020-00529-8

Knutson, D., Soper, J., & Avance, R. (2025). Digital literacy for resistance: Implications for affirming practice with rural TNB youth and their families. *Journal of Health Service Psychology*, *51*(2), 64–71.

Koch, J., & Knutson, D. (2016). Transgender clients in rural areas and small towns. *Journal of Rural Mental Health*, *40*(3–4), 154–163. https://doi.org/10.1037/rmh0000056

Kolhe, C. S., Shikalgar, S., & Biggerstaff, D. (2024). Parental identity and lived experiences when parenting a LGBTQIA+2 child: A critical narrative synthesis of current evidence. *International Journal of Qualitative Studies on Health & Well-Being*, *19*(1), 2738511. https://doi.org/10.1080/17482631.2024.2378511

Lannin, D. G., Vogel, D. L., Guyll, M., & Seidman, A. J. (2019). Reducing threat responses to help-seeking information: Influences of self-affirmations and reassuring information. *Journal of Counseling Psychology*, *66*(3), 375–383. https://doi.org/10.1037/cou0000313

Lawlis, S. M. (2022, January 7). Changing terminology in LGBTQ+ spaces: How to keep up with the lingo. *The Hospitalist*. https://blogs.the-hospitalist.org/content/changing-terminology-lgbtq-spaces-how-keep-lingo

Legato, M. (2020). *The plasticity of sex: The molecular biology and clinical features of genomic sex, gender identity and sexual behavior*. Academic Press.

Leontopoulou, S., & Delle Fave, A. (2022). *Emerging adulthood in the COVID-19 pandemic and other crises: Individual and relational resources*. Springer.

LeVay, S. (2016). *Gay, straight, and the reason why: The science of sexual orientation*. Oxford University Press.

Levine, J. M., Samet, M. G., & Brahlek, R. E. (1975). Information seeking with limitations on available information and resources. *Human Factors*, *17*(5), 502–513.

Lewis, C., & Reynolds, N. (2025). 'Majority doesn't exist': A critical perspective on research with LGBTQ+ people. In *Handbook of sensitive research in the social sciences* (pp. 64–76). Edward Elgar Publishing.

Lind, M., & Thomsen, D. K. (2018). Functions of personal and vicarious life stories: Identity and empathy. *Memory*, *26*(5), 672–682. https://doi.org/10.1080/09658211.2017.1395054

Lindley, L. M., Nagoshi, J. L., Nagoshi, C. T., Hess III, R., & Boscia, A. (2021). An eco-developmental framework on the intersectionality of gender and sexual identities in transgender individuals. *Psychology & Sexuality, 12*(3), 261–278. https://doi.org/10.1080/19419899.2020.1713873

Liu, R. T., & Mustanski, B. (2012). Suicidal ideation and self-harm in lesbian, gay, bisexual, and transgender youth. *American Journal of Preventive Medicine, 42*(3), 221–228. https://doi.org/10.1016/j.amepre.2011.10.023

Magalhães, C. L., Sprott, R. A., & Nic Rider, G. (Eds.). (2022). *Mental health practice with LGBTQ+ children, adolescents, and emerging adults in multiple systems of care.* Rowman & Littlefield.

Martin, C. L., & Fabes, R. A. (2001). The stability and consequences of young children's same-sex peer interactions. *Developmental Psychology, 37*(3), 431–446. https://doi.org/10.1037/0012-1649.37.3.431

Matre, P. J., Dahl, K., Jensen, R., & Nordahl, H. M. (2013). Working with goals in therapy. In E. A. Locke, & G. P. Latham (Eds.), *New developments in goal setting and task performance* (pp.469–490). Routledge.

Matsuno, E., & Israel, T. (2018). Psychological interventions promoting resilience among transgender individuals: Transgender resilience intervention model (TRIM). *The Counseling Psychologist, 46*(5), 632–655.

Matsuno, E., & Israel, T. (2021). The parent support program: Development and acceptability of an online intervention aimed at increasing supportive behaviors among parents of trans youth. *Journal of GLBT Family Studies, 17*(5), 413–431.

Matsuno, E., McConnell, E., Dolan, C. V., & Israel, T. (2022). "I am fortunate to have a transgender child": An investigation into the barriers and facilitators to support among parents of trans and nonbinary youth. *LGBTQ+ Family: An Interdisciplinary Journal, 18*(1), 1–19. https://doi.org/10.1080/1550428X.2021.1991541

Maze, J. R. (2019). *The meaning of behaviour.* Routledge.

McCauley, P. S., Del Farno, A. J., Caba, A. E., Renley, B. M., Shuler, S., Eaton, L. A., & Watson, R. J. (2024). Stress of being outed to parents, LGBTQ family support, and depressive symptoms among sexual and gender diverse youth. *Journal of Research on Adolescence, 34*, 205–221. https://doi.org/10.1111/jora.12912

McConnell, E. A., Birkett, M., & Mustanski, B. (2016). Families matter: Social support and mental health trajectories among lesbian, gay, bisexual, and transgender youth. *Journal of Adolescent Health, 59*(6), 674–680. https://doi.org/10.1016/j.jadohealth.2016.07.026

McLaren, S., Bliss, L. R., Scott, C., Kraidler, P., & Pettignano, R. (2023). Applying a social ecological model to medical legal partnerships practice and research. *Journal of Law, Medicine & Ethics, 51*(4), 817–823. https://doi.org/10.1017/jme.2023.151

Medico, D., Pullen Sansfaçon, A., Zufferey, A., Galantino, G., Bosom, M., & Suerich-Gulick, F. (2020). Pathways to gender affirmation in trans youth: A qualitative and participative study with youth and their parents. *Clinical Child Psychology and Psychiatry, 25*(4), 1002–1014. https://doi.org/10.1177/1359104520938427

Meschke, L. L., Peter, C. R., & Bartholomae, S. (2012). Developmentally appropriate practice to promote healthy adolescent development: Integrating research and practice. *Child & Youth Care Forum, 41*(1), 89–108. https://doi.org/10.1007/s10566-011-9153-7

Milkman, R., Bloom, J., & Narro, V. (2010). *Working for justice: The L.A. model of organizing and advocacy.* Cornell University Press.

Miller, B., & Sprang, G. (2017). A components-based practice and supervision model for reducing compassion fatigue by affecting clinician experience. *Traumatology, 23*(2), 153–164. https://doi.org/10.1037/trm0000058

Mills-Koonce, W. R., Rehder, P. D., & McCurdy, A. L. (2018). The significance of parenting and parent–child relationships for sexual and gender minority adolescents. *Journal of Research on Adolescence, 28(*3), 637–649. https://doi.org/10.1111/jora.12404

Money, L. (2023). Labels and the self: Identity labels as scaffold. *Journal of Analytical Psychology, 68*(3), 590–609. https://doi.org/10.1111/1468-5922.12922

Morgan, H., Heritage, B., Lin, A., Perry, Y., Cook, A., Winter, S., Watson, V., Wright Toussaint, D., O'Donovan, A., Almeida, R., & Strauss, P. (2022). Factors influencing parental acceptance of trans children and young people: Findings from trans pathways. *LGBTQ+ Family: An Interdisciplinary Journal, 18*(5), 475–494. https://doi.org/10.1080/27703371.2022.2125470

Morgan, H., Wells, L., Lin, A., Strauss, P., & Perry, Y. (2023). Parental challenges, facilitators and needs associated with supporting and accepting their trans child's gender. *LGBTQ+ Family: An Interdisciplinary Journal, 19*(1), 70–86. https://doi.org/10.1080/27703371.2022.2142717

Nath, R., Matthews, D., Hobaica, S., Eden, T. M., Taylor, A. B., DeChants, J. P., & Suffredini, K. (2025). *2024 U.S. national survey on the mental health of LGBTQ+ young people by state*. West Hollywood, CA: The Trevor Project. www.thetrevorproject.org/survey-2024-by-state

Neff, K. (2011). *Self-compassion: The proven power of being kind to yourself.* William Morrow.

Newcomb, M. E., Feinstein, B. A., Matson, M., Macapagal, K., & Mustanski, B. (2018). "I have no idea what's going on out there:" Parents' perspectives on promoting sexual health in lesbian, gay, bisexual, and transgender adolescents. *Sexuality Research and Social Policy, 15*(2), 111–122. https://doi.org/10.1007/s13178-018-0326-0

Newman, B. M., & Newman, P. R. (2020). *Theories of adolescent development.* Academic Press.

O'Donohue, W. T., Benuto, L. T., & Tolle, L. W. (2013). *Handbook of adolescent health psychology.* Springer.

Oswald, M. E., & Grosjean, S. (2004). Confirmation bias. *Cognitive Illusions: A Handbook on Fallacies and Biases in Thinking, Judgement and Memory, 79*, 83.

Post, G. (2025). Resilient parents; resilient kids: How parental self-awareness is critical to helping smart kids thrive. *Gifted Education International, 41*(1), 92–111. https://doi.org/10.1177/02614294241274442

Prochaska, J. O., & DiClemente, C. C. (1983). Stages and processes of self-change of smoking: Toward an integrative model of change. *Journal of Consulting and Clinical Psychology, 51*(3), 390–395. https://doi.org/10.1037//0022-006x.51.3.390

Pullen Sansfaçon, A., Medico, D., Suerich-Gulick, F., & Temple Newhook, J. (2020). "I knew that I wasn't cis, I knew that, but I didn't know exactly": Gender identity development, expression and affirmation in youth who access gender affirming medical care. *International Journal of Transgender Health, 21*(3), 307–320. https://doi.org/10.1080/26895269.2020.1756551

Pullen Sansfaçon, A., Robichaud, M. J., & Dumais-Michaud, A.-A. (2015). The experience of parents who support their children's gender variance. *Journal of LGBT Youth, 12*(1), 39–63. https://doi.org/10.1080/19361653.2014.935555

Rainbow, C., Tatnell, R., Blashki, G., Fuller-Tyszkiewicz, M., & Melvin, G. A. (2024). Digital safety plan effectiveness and use: Findings from a three-month longitudinal study. *Psychiatry Research, 333*. https://doi.org/10.1016/j.psychrs.2024.115748

Ratts, M. J., Singh, A. A., Nassar-McMillan, S., Butler, S. K., & McCullough, J. R. (2016). Multicultural and social justice counseling competencies: Guidelines for the counseling profession. *Journal of Multicultural Counseling and Development, 44*(1), 28–48. https://doi.org/10.1002/jmcd.12035

Ream, G. L. (2022). Trends in deaths by suicide 2014–2019 among lesbian, gay, bisexual, transgender, queer, questioning, and other gender/sexual minority (LGBTQ+) youth. *Journal of Adolescent Health, 71*(5), 609–615. https://doi.org/10.1016/j.jadohealth.2022.06.017

Riesch, S. K., Anderson, L. S., & Krueger, H. A. (2006). Parent–child communication processes: Preventing children's health-risk behavior. *Journal for Specialists in Pediatric Nursing, 11*(1), 41–56. https://doi.org/10.1111/j.1744-6155.2006.00042.x

Roe, S. (2017). "Family support would have been like amazing": LGBTQ youth experiences with parental and family support. *The Family Journal, 25*(1), 55–62. https://doi.org/10.1177/1066480716679651

Rogers, M. L., Gai, A. R., Lieberman, A., Musacchio Schafer, K., & Joiner, T. E. (2022). Why does safety planning prevent suicidal behavior? *Professional Psychology: Research and Practice, 53*(1), 33–41. https://doi.org/10.1037/pro0000427

Rosenzweig, S. (1936). Some implicit common factors in diverse methods of psychotherapy. *American Journal of Orthopsychiatry, 6*(3), 412–415. https://doi.org/10.1111/j.1939-0025.1936.tb05248.x

Roskam, I., Gross, J. J., & Mikolajczak, M. (Eds.). (2023). *Emotion regulation and parenting.* Cambridge University Press.

Rossi, A. L., & Lopez, E. J. (2017). Contextualizing competence: Language and LGBT-based competency in health care. *Journal of Homosexuality, 64*(10), 1330–1349. https://doi.org/10.1080/00918369.2017.1321361

Roughgarden, J. (2013). *Evolution's rainbow: Diversity, gender, and sexuality in nature and people* (1st ed.). University of California Press.

Rutherford, H. J. V. (2023). Neurobiology of parenting and implications for emotion regulation. In I. Roskam, J. J. Gross, & M. Mikolajczak (Eds.), *Emotion regulation and parenting* (pp. 229–243). Cambridge University Press.

Ryan, C., & Chen-Hayes, S. F. (2013). Educating and empowering families of lesbian, gay, bisexual, transgender, and questioning students. In E. S. Fisher, & K. Komosa-Hawkins (Eds.), *Creating safe and supportive learning environments* (pp. 209–229). Routledge.

Ryan, C., Huebner, D., Diaz, R. M., & Sanchez, J. (2009). Family rejection as a predictor of negative health outcomes in white and latino lesbian, gay, and bisexual young adults. *Pediatrics, 123*(1), 346–352. https://doi.org/10.1542/peds.2007-3524

Saenz, A. (2015). *Relationships that work: Four ways to connect (and set boundaries) with colleagues, students, and parents*. Routledge.

Salgado, D. M., White, A. W., Peterson, D., & Dimeff, L. A. (2019). Cultivating wise mind in dialectical behavior therapy through mindfulness. In I. Ivtzan (Ed.), *Handbook of mindfulness-based programmes*. Routledge.

Satinover, J. (1996). The gay gene. *The Journal of Human Sexuality, 1*, 3–10.

Scherer, K. R. (2005). Unconscious processes in emotion: The bulk of the iceberg. In L. F. Barrett, P. M. Niedenthal, & P. Winkielman (Eds.), *Emotion and consciousness* (pp. 312–334). The Guilford Press.

Schneider, N. (2021). Stigmatization. In *Encyclopedia of autism spectrum disorders* (pp. 4635–4636). Cham: Springer International Publishing.

Schultz, K., Cattaneo, L. B., Sabina, C., Brunner, L., Jackson, S., & Serrata, J. V. (2016). Key roles of community connectedness in healing from trauma. *Psychology of Violence, 6*(1), 42–48. https://doi.org/10.1037/vio0000025

Siegel, D. J., & Payne Bryson, T. (2011). *The whole-brain child: 12 revolutionary strategies to nurture your child's developing mind*. Bantam Books.

Singer, J. L., & Pope, K. S. (2012). The use of imagery and fantasy techniques in psychotherapy. In J. L. Singer, & K. S. Pope (Eds.), *The power of human imagination: New methods in psychotherapy* (pp. 3–34). Springer.

Sommer, V., & Vasey, P. L. (2006). Homosexual behaviour in animals: Topics, hypotheses and research trajectories. In V. Sommer, & P. L. Vasey (Eds.), *Homosexual behaviour in animals: An evolutionary perspective* (pp. 3–42). Cambridge University Press.

Springer, K. S., & Tolin, D. F. (2020). *The big book of exposures*. New Harbinger Publications.

Tarantino, M. R., & Jamison, T. B. (2023). Resilience through relationship experiences: A qualitative exploration of lesbian, gay, and bisexual romantic development. *LGBTQ+ Family: An Interdisciplinary Journal, 19*(5), 351–366. https://doi.org/10.1080/27703371.2023.2212621

Tate, D. P., & Patterson, C. J. (2019). Sexual orientation, relationships with parents, stress, and depressive symptoms among adults. *Journal of GLBT Family Studies, 15*(3), 256–271. https://doi.org/10.1080/1550428X.2018.1486263

Testa, R. J., Habarth, J., Peta, J., Balsam, K., & Bockting, W. (2015). Development of the gender minority stress and resilience measure. *Psychology of Sexual Orientation and Gender Diversity, 2*(1), 65–77. https://doi.org/10.1037/sgd0000081

Thomsen, D. K., & Pillemer, D. B. (2017). I know my story and i know your story: Developing a conceptual framework for vicarious life stories. *Journal of Personality, 85*(4), 464–480. https://doi.org/10.1111/jopy.12253

Tsvieli, N., Nir, G. O., Lifshitz, C., Diamond, G. S., Kobak, R., & Diamond, G. M. (2020). Therapist interventions associated with productive emotional processing in the context of attachment based family therapy for depressed and suicidal adolescents. *Family Process, 59*(2), 428–444. https://doi.org/10.1111/famp.12445

Urban, B., Knutson, D., Klooster, D., & Soper, J. (2022). Social-contextual influences on eating pathology in transgender and nonbinary adults. *Eating Disorders: The Journal of Treatment and Prevention*. https://doi.org/10.1080/10640266.2022.2135715

Urmanche, A. A., Oliveira, J. T., Gonçalves, M. M., Eubanks, C. F., & Muran, J. C. (2019). Ambivalence, resistance, and alliance ruptures in psychotherapy: It's complicated. *Psychoanalytic Psychology, 36*(2), 139–147. https://doi.org/10.1037/pap0000237

van Bergen, D. D., Wilson, B. D. M., Russell, S. T., Gordon, A. G., & Rothblum, E. D. (2021). Parental responses to coming out by lesbian, gay, bisexual, queer, pansexual, or two-spirited people across three age cohorts. *Journal of Marriage and Family, 83*(4), 1116–1133. https://doi.org/10.1111/jomf.12731

Van Orden, K. A., Witte, T. K., Cukrowicz, K. C., Braithwaite, S. R., Selby, E. A., & Joiner Jr., T. E. (2010). The interpersonal theory of suicide. *Psychological Review, 117*(2), 575–600. https://doi.org/10.1037/a0018697

Vaughan, M. D., & Rodriguez, E. M. (2014). LGBT strengths: Incorporating positive psychology into theory, research, training, and practice. *Psychology of Sexual Orientation and Gender Diversity, 1*(4), 325–334. https://doi.org/10.1037/sgd0000053

Walker, A. (2018). *Collective consciousness and gender*. Palgrave Macmillan UK. https://doi.org/10.1057/978-1-137-54414-8

Wells, K., & McCaig, M. (2016). The magic wand question and recovery-focused practice in child and adolescent mental health services. *Journal of Child and Adolescent Psychiatric Nursing, 29*(4), 164–170. https://doi.org/10.1111/jcap.12159

Whittingham, K., & Coyne, L. W. (2019). Values and proto-values. In K. Whittingham, & L. W. Coyne (Eds.), *Acceptance and commitment therapy* (pp. 153–186). Academic Press.

Whittlesey, C. (2022). *The beginner's guide to being a trans ally*. Jessica Kingsley Publishers.

Wilkes, R., & Wu, C. (2018). Trust and minority groups. In E. M. Uslaner (Ed.), *The oxford handbook of social and political trust* (pp. 231–250). Oxford University Press.

Willner, G. (1968). The role of anxiety in obsessivecompulsive disorders. *The American Journal of Psychoanalysis, 28*(1), 201–211.

Wilson, K. G., & Murrell, A. R. (2011). Values work in acceptance and commitment therapy. In S. C. Hayes, V. M. Follette, & M. M. Linehan (Eds.), *Mindfulness and acceptance: Expanding the cognitive-behavioral tradition*. Guilford Press.

World Health Organization. (2023, December 1). *Human rights*. https://www.who.int/news-room/fact-sheets/detail/human-rights-and-health

Yep, G. A. (2021). From being to doing: Toward a reconceptualization of LGBTQ worldmaking allies. *QED: A Journal in GLBTQ Worldmaking, 8*(2), 75–80. https://www.jstor.org/stable/48655678

Zaki, J. (2020). Integrating empathy and interpersonal emotion regulation. *Annual Review of Psychology, 71*, 517–540. https://doi.org/10.1146/annurev-psych-010419-050830

INDEX